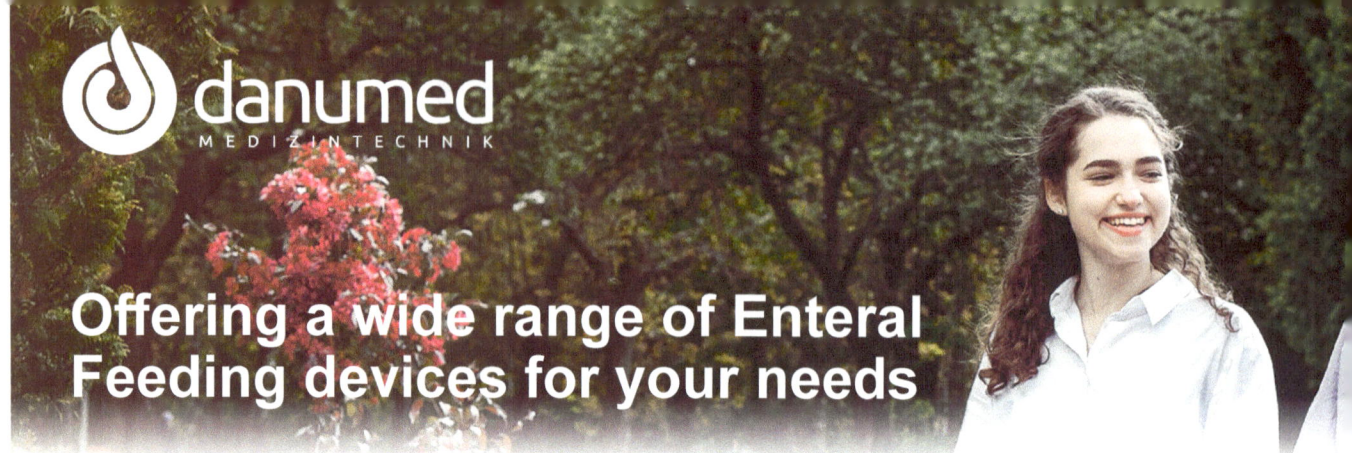

Offering a wide range of Enteral Feeding devices for your needs

Increasing Comfort and Safety
danuButton®

The danuButton® is a replacement feeding tube for long-term enteral nutrition and use with a completely healed stomas.

The right danuButton® for every patient

✓ Variety of sizes and lengths

Small, low in profile and discreet

✓ Easily hidden under clothing, allows for the best possible freedom of movement

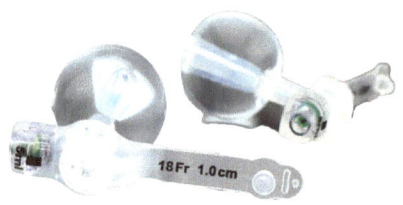

High-quality materials for safety and comfort

✓ danuButton® is very soft and flexible for excellent wearing comfort

✓ Latex-free, PVC-free, free of harmful plasticisers such as DEHP or BPA

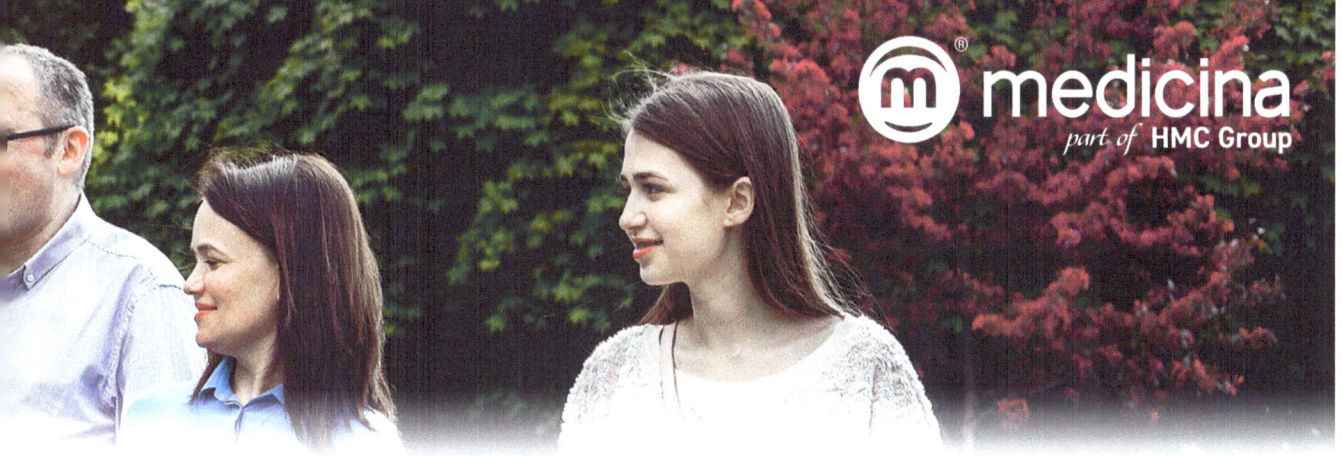

At Home ENFit Reusable Syringes

The ENFit Reusable range of enteral syringes has been developed to deliver enteral feeds, medicines and flushes safely to neonatal, paediatric and adult patients at home.

Enhancing patient safety

Features

✓ Reusable/Washable

✓ Individually packaged

✓ Customer support

✓ Clear measurement markings

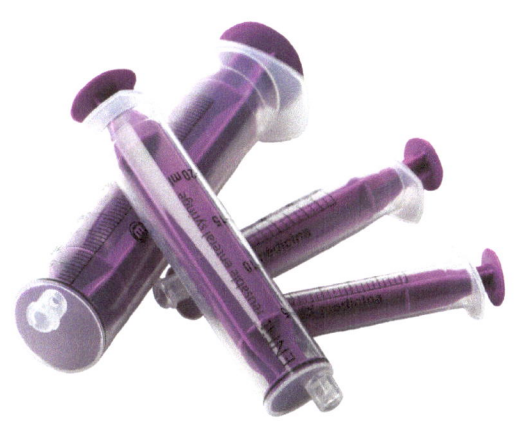

ALWAYS READ THE LABEL AND FOLLOW DIRECTIONS FOR USE. Consult your healthcare professional to see which product is right for you. AMSL is a subsidiary of Dexcom

For more information on the Medicina and danumed range, please contact us on **(02) 9882 3666** or at **amsl@amsl.com.au**

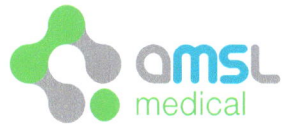

amsl.com.au

Australasian Medical and Scientific Ltd. 2 McCabe Place, Chatswood, NSW 2097.

The Blend Issue Two was created in partnership with...

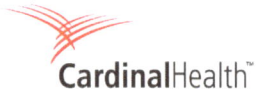 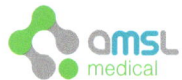 **AVANOS**

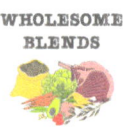 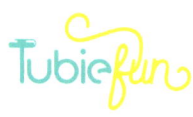

whole enteral 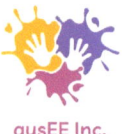 EVERYHUMAN

the blend.

Disclaimer
This resource is for general information and support purposes only. The information is not intended as a substitute for professional medical advice and if you have questions or concerns regarding your health or that of your child, please seek assistance from a qualified and licensed health professional. While every effort is made to ensure that the information contained in this book is accurate and appropriate, *The Blend* creators make no warranty of any kind, expressed or implied, and are not liable for the accuracy, currency, errors or omissions in the information contained here. All access to, and use of, the information is at the reader's discretion and risk.

Credits
The Blend is curated, written and edited by Melanie Dimmitt and designed by Edie Swan. Issue Two's cover star is Loretta Harmes, photographed by Amy Maidment. Much of the recipe nutritional analysis was done, very kindly, by Kate Dehlsen.

Acknowledgement of Country
The Blend creators acknowledge the Aboriginal and Torres Strait Islander peoples of Australia. We acknowledge the Gundungurra, Tharawal and Garigal peoples, the traditional custodians of the lands on which *The Blend* was made. We pay our respects to ancestors and Elders, both past, present and emerging.

the blend.
contents

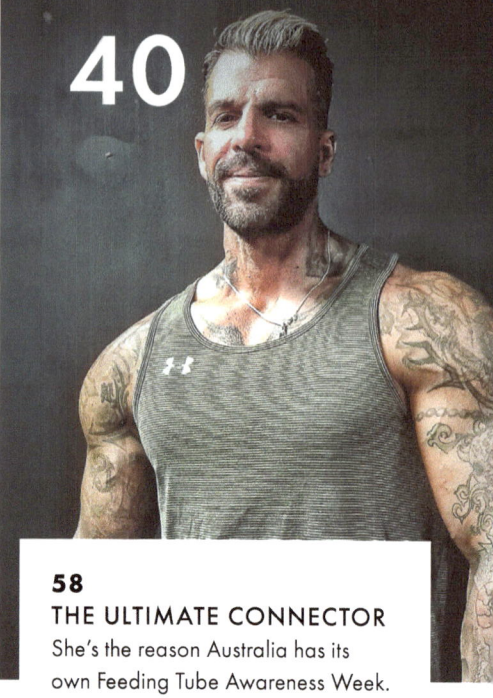
40

09
Glossary

10
Editor's letter

20
Five minutes with the makers
Catch up with the tube-feeding mothers and business mavericks behind Tubie Fun, Miracle Mumma, Whole Enteral and Wholesome Blends.

Personal accounts

26
CHRONICALLY CREATIVE
A bout of maternal sepsis shook her world. But amid the medical chaos, Megan Fisher has found beauty.

32
ACQUIRED TASTE
What's it like to eat your first chip sandwich in your late teens? Mind blowing. Just ask Alexander Vane.

40
STRONG STOMACH
With a body that screams power and a G-tube in place, Pedro Relvas is annihilating assumptions.

Professional perspectives

50
THE SEASONED EXPERT
Hilarie Dreyer is a dietitian on a mission to help families master tube-feeding at home.

54
THE GUT HEALER
Paediatric gastroenterologist Usha Krishnan shares how blenderised tube-feeds are taking off and taming troubled tummies.

58
THE ULTIMATE CONNECTOR
She's the reason Australia has its own Feeding Tube Awareness Week. Sarah Gray, the founder of ausEE Inc., reflects on the importance of community.

Cover story

66
THE NIL BY MOUTH FOODIE
Loretta Harmes can't eat another bite. Literally. Nevertheless, her culinary talent and incredible story has made her a star.

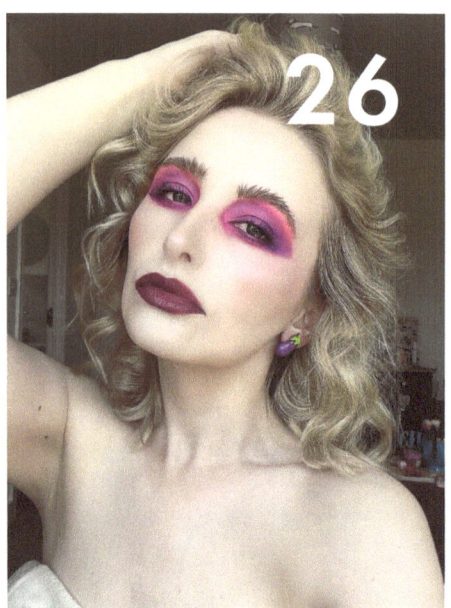
26

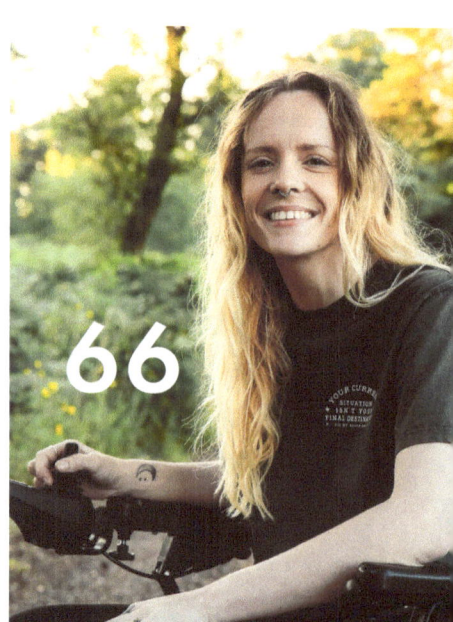
66

Parent stories

76
TUBIE TRUTHS
Nina Alhambra has learnt that, when it comes to what's right for her daughter, Mama really does know best.

82
SMASHING IT
Why let a tube hold you back? Eliana Joseph makes sure her family doesn't miss out on a moment of fun.

88
POST-TRAUMATIC PRIDE
Host of The Rare Life podcast, Madeline Cheney, shares a personal essay on the emotional agony – and epic bravery – of tube-feeding a newborn.

92
A LOVE LIKE NO OTHER
Meet Brana Gadsby and Ross Worth, parents who are shouting their daughter's worth and changing the way the world looks at tube-feeding families.

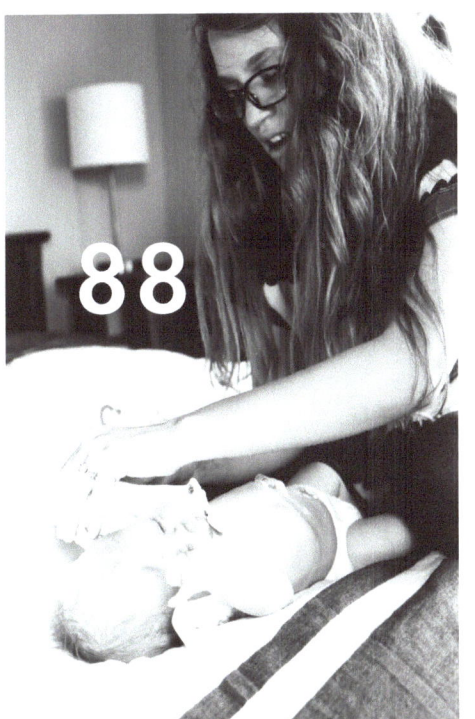

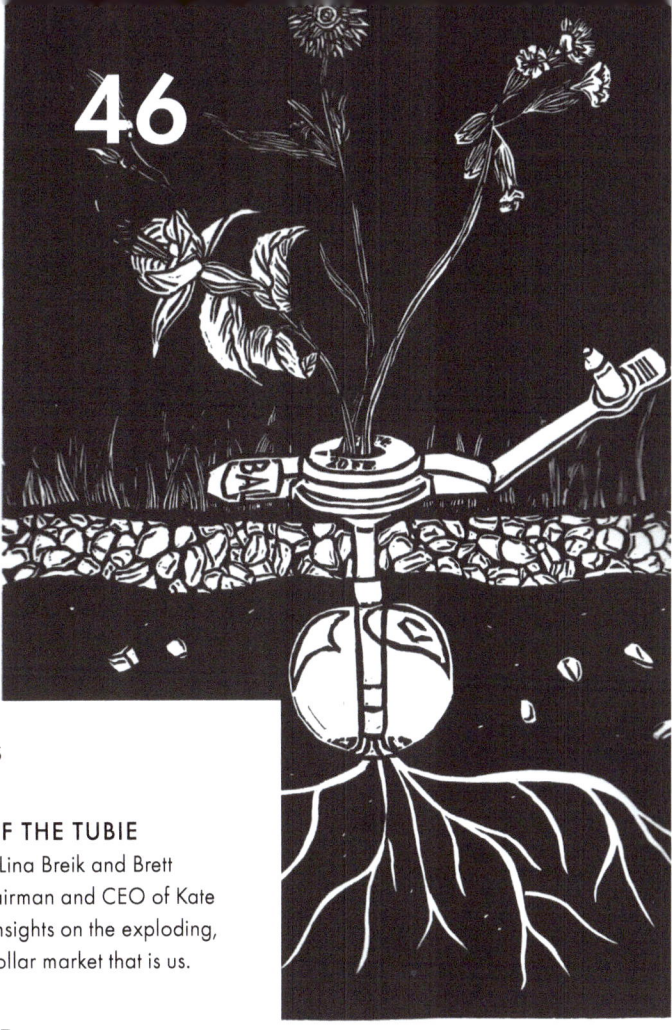

Features

12
THE AGE OF THE TUBIE
Tube Dietitian Lina Breik and Brett Matthews, chairman and CEO of Kate Farms, share insights on the exploding, multi-billion-dollar market that is us.

36
TUBIE TO BE
Kate Thomas will eventually start tube-feeding, so she did what any good journalist would do – hunted down primary sources who were experienced tube-feeders and (politely) probed them.

46
G-TUBE FEEDING 101
Expert tips for getting a grip on a gastrostomy (G) tube from Robyn Wortel, a specialist who teaches doctors about tube-feeding.

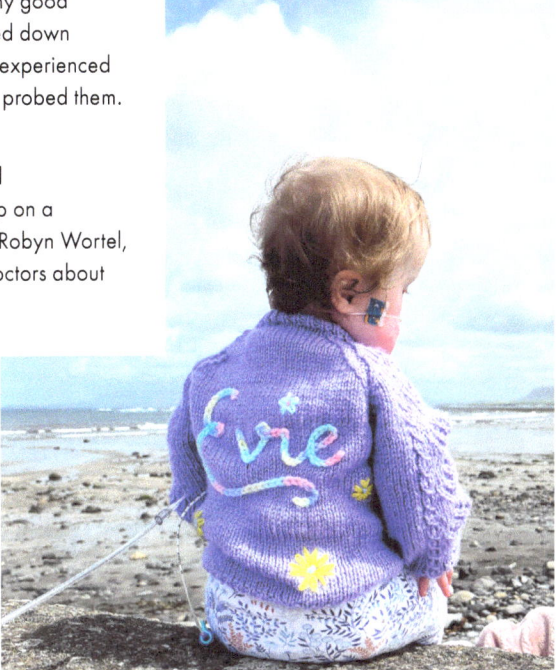

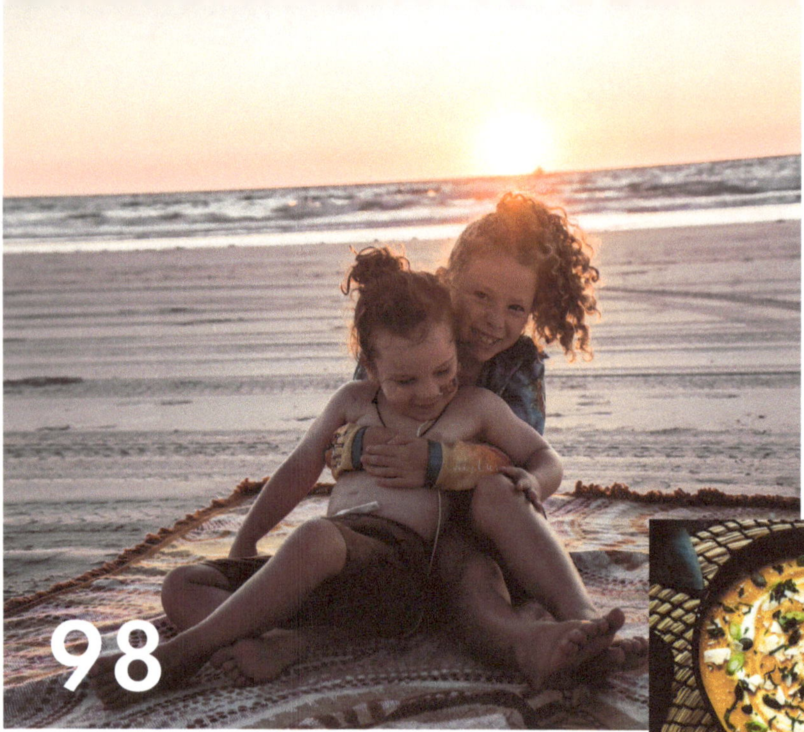

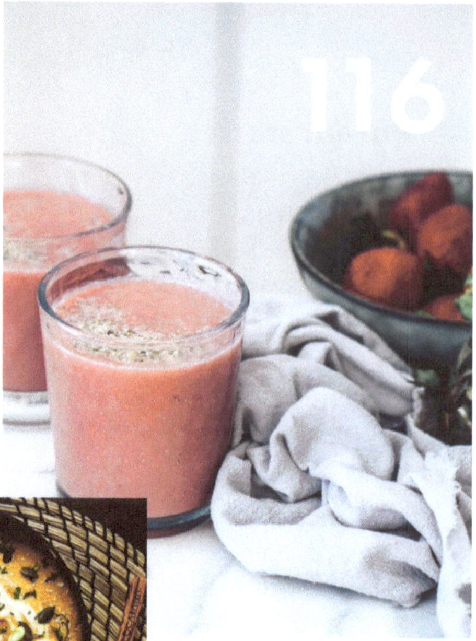

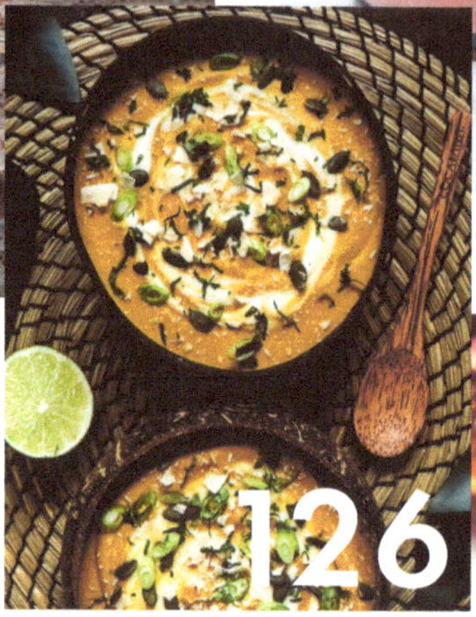

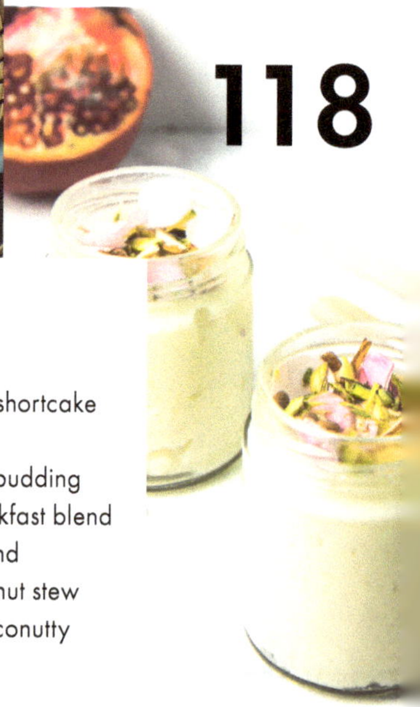

Features continued...

64
ARTIST IN RESIDENCE
Tube-fed creative Kathryn Lean shares some of her latest works.

98
TRAVELLING TUBIE
Think you can't adventure with a feeding tube? Think again. Get wanderlusting over Chloe Turner's story of caravanning around the country with her family.

Recipes

116 Hilarie Dreyer's strawberry shortcake overnight oats
118 Lina Breik's rose water milk pudding
120 Kate Dehlsen's English breakfast blend
122 Sarah Thomas's nachos blend
124 Claire Kariya's African peanut stew
126 Loretta Harmes' roasted coconutty butternut squash soup

Directory

128
A collection of products and online communities for tube-feeding.

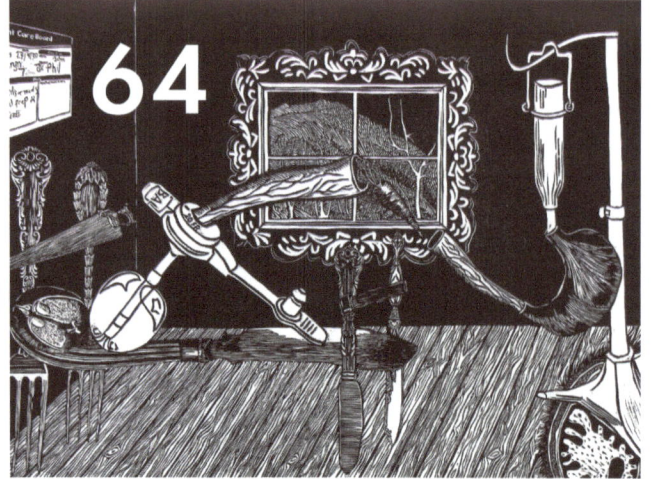

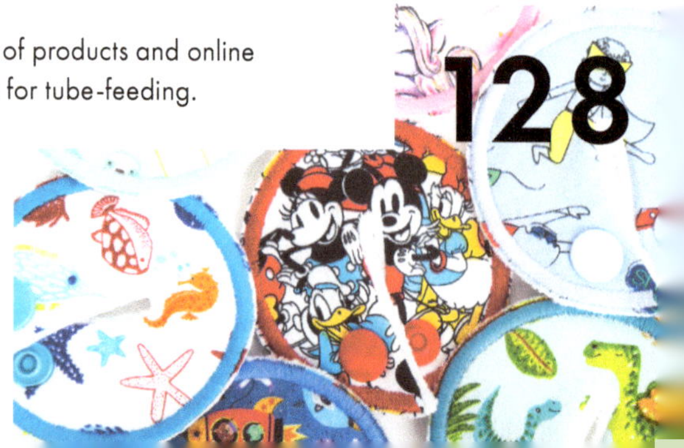

Glossary

ADHD (attention-deficit/hyperactivity disorder) is a neurodevelopmental condition characterised by heightened levels of inattention, impulsivity and hyperactivity.

Anaphylaxis is a severe, potentially life-threatening allergic reaction that requires urgent treatment with adrenaline (epinephrine).

Aspiration means accidentally inhaling liquid or food into the windpipe and/or lungs.

Blenderised food or a **blenderised diet** is real food, blended with liquid and put through a feeding tube.

Bolus feeding means large amounts of formula delivered through the tube.

Continuous feeding means feeding small amounts of formula constantly throughout the day (or night) without interruption.

Ehlers-Danlos syndrome (EDS) is a group of inherited connective tissue disorders mainly affecting the joints, skin and walls of blood vessels.

Enteral feeding is a method of supplying nutrients directly into the gastrointestinal tract.

Epilepsy is a chronic neurological disorder characterised by the tendency to have recurrent seizures.

A **feeding pump** is a small, plug-in or battery powered machine that automatically controls the amount of formula being delivered through the feeding tube.

A **gastrostomy** is a surgical opening (stoma) through the skin into the stomach.

A **gastrostomy (G) tube** is placed through the skin of the abdomen straight to the stomach.

A **gastrostomy-jejunostomy (G-J) tube** is placed into the stomach and small intestine.

A **giving set** is tubing that connects the feeding container to the feeding tube.

Granulation tissue is fleshy projections formed on the surface of the stoma.

A **jejunostomy (J) tube** is placed through the skin of the abdomen straight into the intestines.

Mast cell activation syndrome (MCAS) is a condition that causes the body's mast cells (a type of white blood cell found in connective tissues) to release too much of a substance that causes allergy-like symptoms.

Microbiome are the microorganisms in a particular environment including the body or a part of the body, for example, the intestinal tract.

A **nasogastric (NG) tube** starts in the nose and ends in the stomach.

A **nasojejunal (NJ) tube** passes through the nose and into the small bowel.

The **NDIS** is Australia's National Disability Insurance Scheme.

The **newborn intensive care unit (NICU)** is a hospital intensive care unit that specialises in looking after premature and unwell newborn babies.

A **percutaneous endoscopic gastrostomy (PEG)** is a surgery to place a feeding tube.

Post-traumatic stress disorder (PTSD) is a form of anxiety disorder that's triggered by either experiencing or witnessing a terrifying event.

A **stoma** is a surgical opening through which a feeding tube can enter the body.

A **tonic-clonic seizure**, also called a grand mal seizure, is a type of seizure involving a loss of consciousness and violent muscle contractions.

Total parenteral nutrition (TPN) is complete nutrition delivered intravenously (directly into a person's vein), bypassing the gastrointestinal tract.

A **tracheostomy** is an opening created at the front of the neck so a tube can be inserted into the windpipe (trachea) to help you breathe.

Venting means letting gas from a person's stomach out through the end of their G-tube to remove excess air and relieve fullness and bloating.

A message from the editor, Melanie Dimmitt

Photography: Abbie Melle

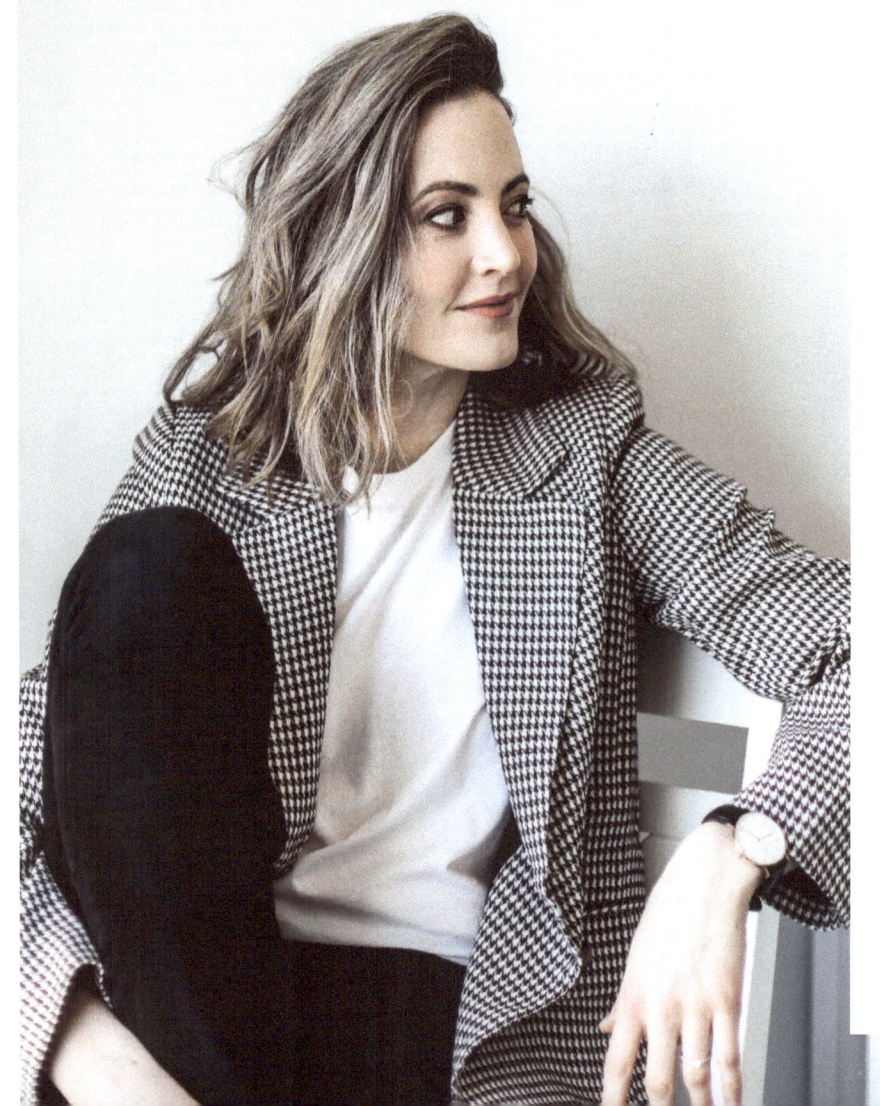

So, it's been a year. And somehow, a magazine for tube-feeders has made enough of a splash to get itself a second issue. Thank you to the sponsors, contributors and readers who've made this possible. Welcome again, friends, to The Blend.

Congratulations are in order as we've seen huge progress on the tube-feeding front. Back in 2021, a bunch of experts put their heads together and created an evidence-based guide to blended feeds for clinicians in Australia and New Zealand. Known as 'the consensus statement', that guide has really caught on.

As a result, the medical sector's attitude toward this diet is shifting from 'nope, no can do' to 'how can we support you?'. Read more about this and other exciting, global enteral-feeding developments in our feature, The Age of the Tubie, on page 12.

/ **editor's letter**

Never before have tube-feeders had so much choice over what sustains them, but as the Covid pandemic persists, they've also faced enormous challenges.

Our community has been rocked by worldwide product shortages. We've experienced major delivery delays, with certain formulas and equipment all but impossible to get a hold of. It's been heartening to see social media networks band together during this time, sending precious supplies to people and families in need.

Despite this ongoing issue, the global enteral feeding market is booming and set to reach close to $US10 billion by the end of the decade. And while we're in the realm of extremely large numbers, there are more than a billion TikTok videos attached to the hashtag #feedingtube. You'll meet Cyprus-based TikTok tube-feeding star, Deren Kıralp, in a story by soon-to-be tubie and journalist Kate Thomas, on page 36.

In my own small patch of this space I've made a life-changing discovery: reusable syringes! The ones with silicone O-rings are immeasurably better than your stock-standard, single-use variety for blended feeds. Not to mention less guilt-inducing on the wastage front.

In other news, under the careful supervision of nurses at our local hospital, I changed my now six-year-old son Arlo's MIC-KEY button all by myself. Yep, I did it. And implore other tubie parents to give it a go.

Like many humans on this planet, our family all got Covid in the year just gone. Arlo sailed through it more smoothly than his medically boring family members – in no small part due, I'm sure, to his G-tube keeping aspiration off the menu. I join many other people on the pages to come in saying, thank frick for that tube.

It's been an absolute treat to gather stories for this issue of The Blend. We've gone more global this time, so prepare to soak in wisdom from tube-feeding people, families and professionals the world over.

"If you take just one message from this magazine, let it be that you are not alone."

Read compelling words from The Nil By Mouth Foodie, our cover star, and an extraordinary tale from The Chronic Makeup Artist. Go adventuring with a tubie family caravanning around Australia. Be moved by a heart-wrenching essay from the host of The Rare Life podcast, buoyed by parents who are shouting their child's worth, and inspired by a tube-feeding bodybuilder who'd out-muscle Arnie.

If you take just one message from this magazine, let it be that you are not alone. We are a big, creative and caring community, celebrating this way of eating and living full, beautiful lives.

Much love,

Mel xx

melaniedimmitt.com.au
theblendmag.com
@the_special_book

the blend.

Rate = Volume ÷ Time, 2022
Linocut Print on Paper, 21x29cm

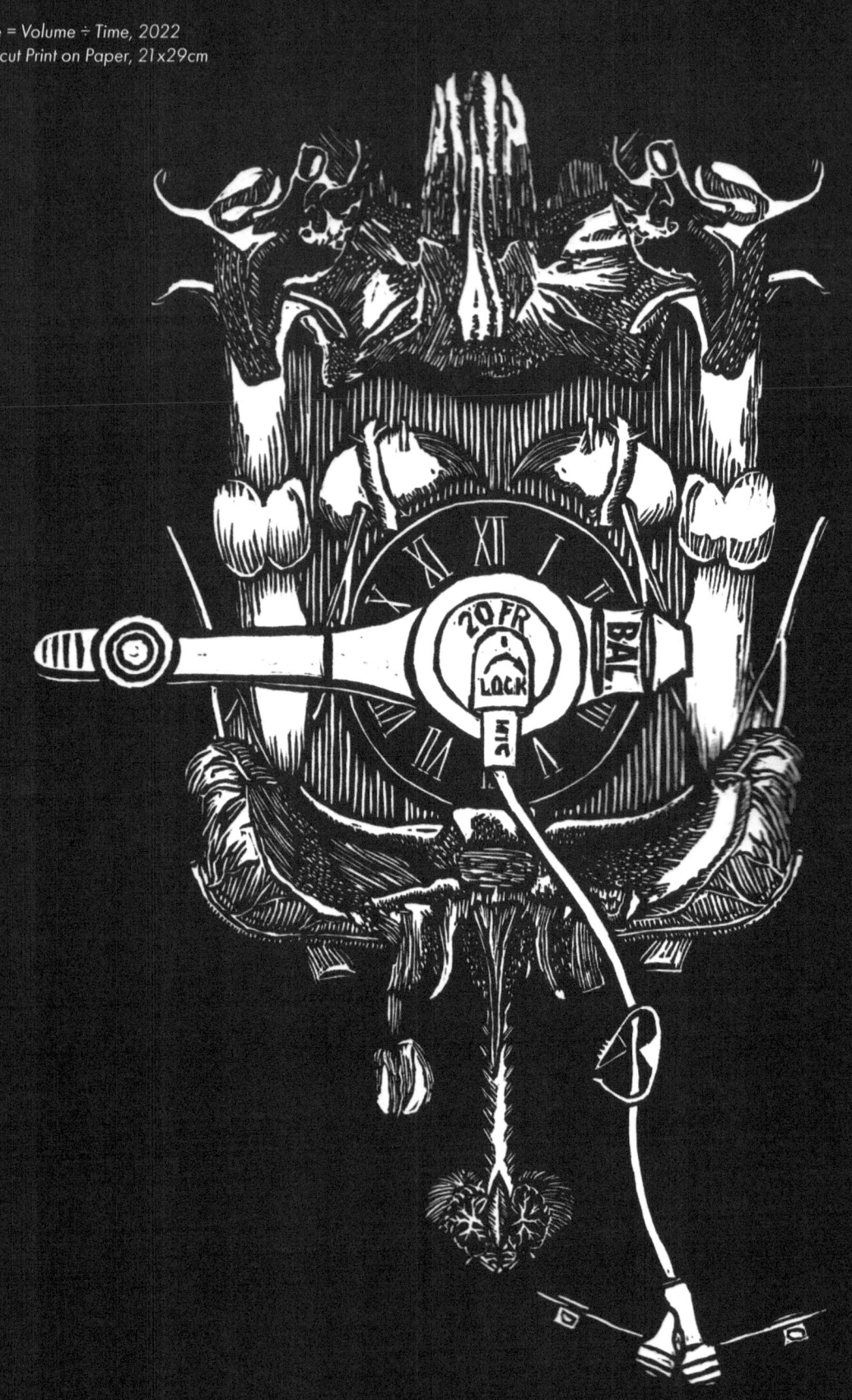

/ feature

The age of the tubie

Think you're in a niche? News flash: You're not. The global tube-feeding community is growing, getting attention and giving the medical sector a much-needed shake-up.

Artwork: Kathryn Lean

There's never been a better time to be tube-fed. Not only because a century ago, tube-feeders received nutrition through a decidedly unappetising orifice*. But also due to the fact that we, the tube-feeding community of today, are a booming market. We have a rising voice and we're demanding better.

Not long ago, the first issue of this magazine was described as 'radical' by a professional in the paediatric feeding space. That professional is pro-choice when it comes to what their patients put down their tubes, but all the same, they were extremely careful to detach from the major hospital they worked for while discussing blended feeds.

Up until very recently, this diet was controversial.

For decades, the vast majority of the medical sector has prescribed a limited range of commercial formulas for tube-feeders. But in the privacy of home kitchens, people were blitzing forbidden fruit, vegetables, meats, grains and dairy – even the occasional slice of cake – on the sly.

Things started to change when, in July 2021, the Australasian Society of Parenteral and Enteral Nutrition (AuSPEN) released its blended tube-feeding consensus statement, a seven-page document neatly summarising the current research and expert clinical opinions around enteral blended tube feeds. >>

*Read Issue One of The Blend for a short history of tube-feeding in all its rectal-feeding glory.

the blend.   13

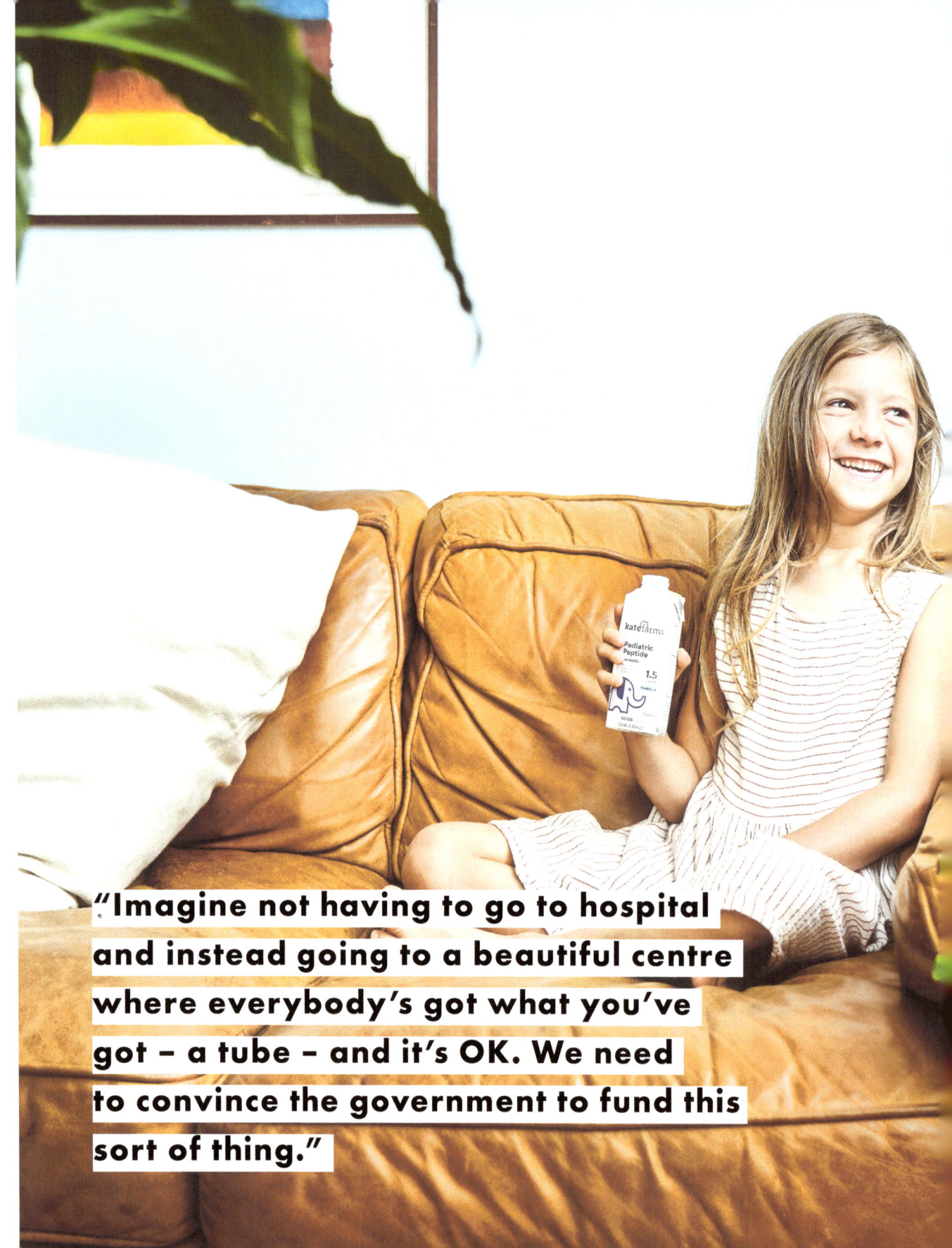

"Imagine not having to go to hospital and instead going to a beautiful centre where everybody's got what you've got – a tube – and it's OK. We need to convince the government to fund this sort of thing."

/ feature

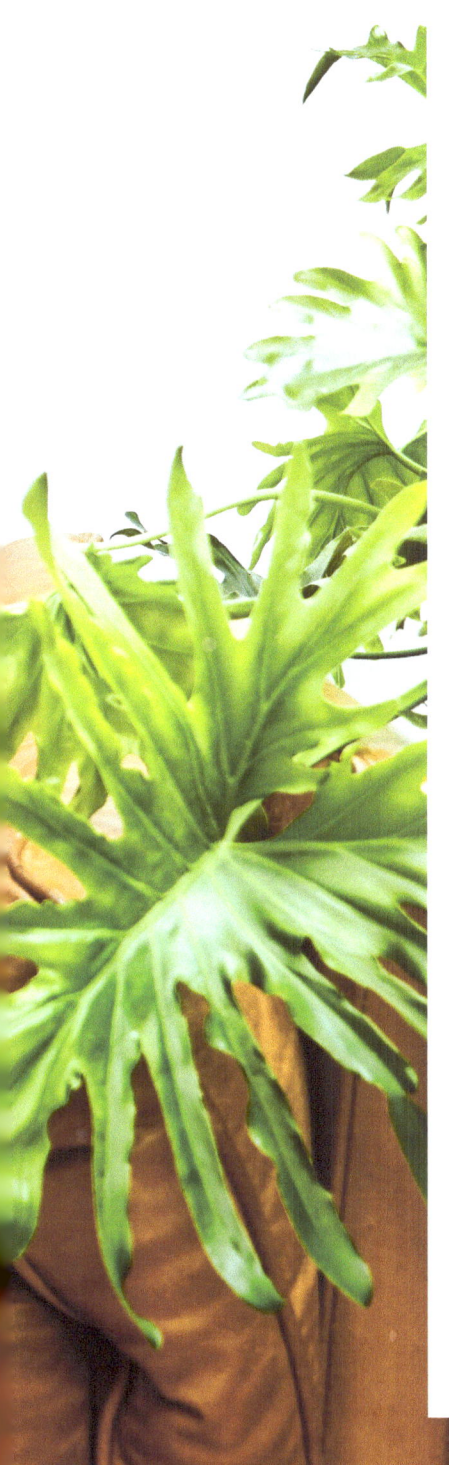

No longer was this diet shrouded in doubt and questions like, should we be doing it? Is it safe? Does it block tubes?

'That's all changed to asking, what should we recommend?, which is really brilliant,' says Lina Breik, a senior dietitian with a particular passion for helping people tube-feed. Known professionally as the Tube Dietitian, Lina marvels over this refreshing reference for medical professionals, describing the general vibe of the AuSPEN statement as 'extremely positive'.

'It's very much about autonomy, independence and people's choice and I think that's where the shift is happening,' says Lina. 'Tube-fed nutrition – especially in the home – is no longer a medical thing. And it shouldn't be. Nutrition in the home is about love, connection and culture.'

Baffled by the lack of existing data around Australians who tube-feed, Lina has decided to spend three years gathering stories from this community as part of her PhD.

'I want to hear about people's experiences,' Lina explains. 'Say you're a 40-year-old person who's had a stroke and now needs a feeding tube. You're at a cafe with your friends, everyone's tucking into their meal and you're there with your tube. Do you feel welcome? Do you feel comfortable whipping out your bolus syringe? Do we need to have tubie-friendly stickers in cafes so people with tubes can feel comfortable feeding in public?'

Lina dreams of a day when every Australian city has its own tube-feeding hub, where people can come together and access experienced specialists.

'Imagine not having to go to hospital and instead going to a beautiful centre where everybody's got what you've got – a tube – and it's OK,' she says. 'We need to convince the government to fund this sort of thing and for that, we need data. I'm hoping to start the process of collecting information on who's in this community and how they're feeling.'

A decade ago, Brett Matthews was feeling desperate. His teenage son, Skyler, was getting progressively sicker and his doctors couldn't figure out why.

'They were going to put him on chemotherapy – for an autoimmune disease – and that just didn't feel right,' Brett recalls. 'We were searching for solutions and met some amazing registered dietitians and naturopaths who, through nutrition alone, got Skyler on a path of healing.'

Brett is now the chairman and chief executive of Kate Farms, a US company producing organic, plant-based formulas that started because an unwell girl had parents who, like Brett, weren't willing to accept the status quo.

'I met Richard and Michelle Laver and their daughter, Kate, who was born with cerebral palsy,' he says. 'At five years old Kate was severely underweight. She got a feeding tube, but her body couldn't process the synthetic formulas available to her.' >>

the blend.

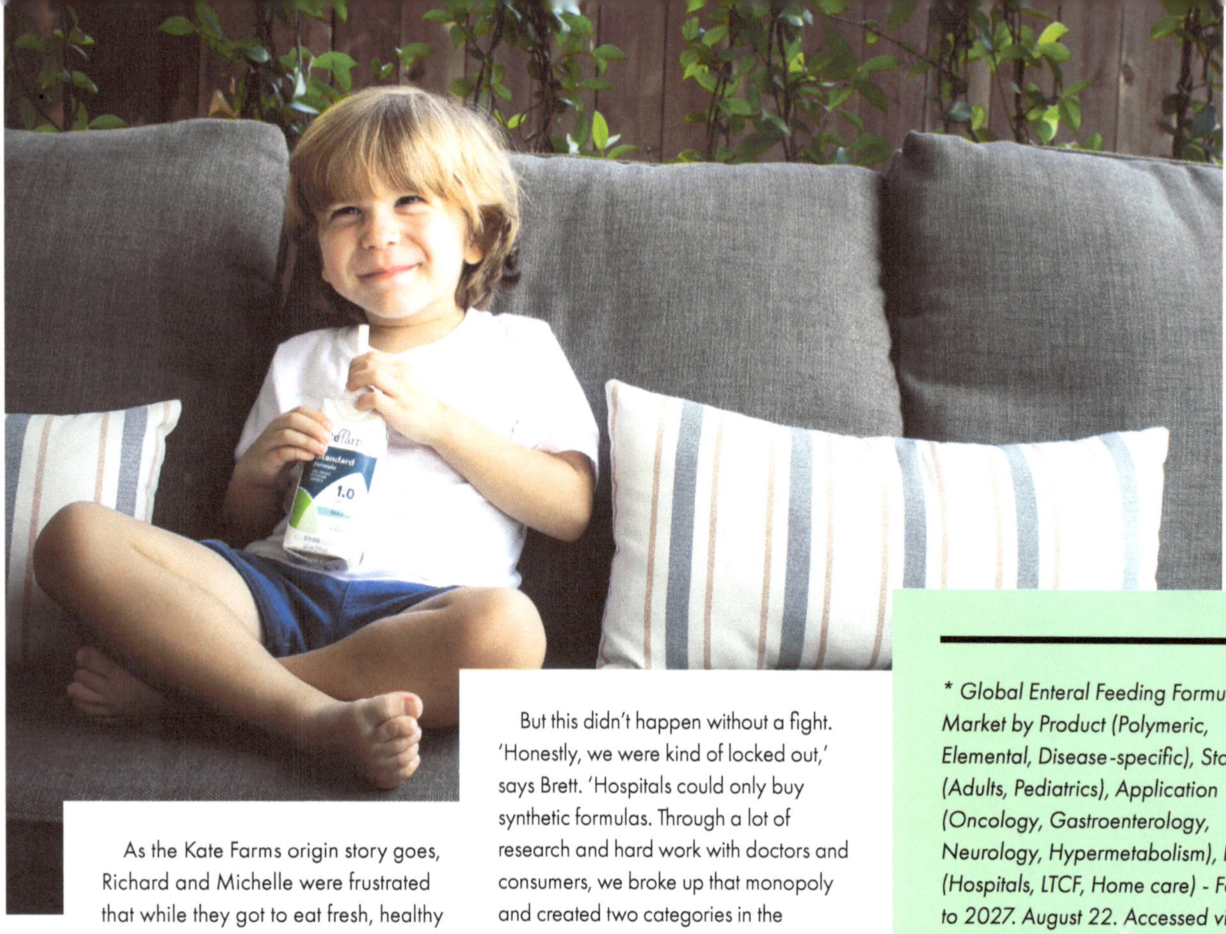

As the Kate Farms origin story goes, Richard and Michelle were frustrated that while they got to eat fresh, healthy food, Kate was forced to make do with formulas made of sugar, corn syrup and emulsifiers. So they raided their local organic grocery store, revved up their blender and, after trialling 70 different recipes, number 71 saw Kate's health dramatically improve.

'She just turned 16 and she's thriving,' says Brett – and so is the business that she inspired.

Last September, Kate Farms raised $US75 million in its Series C round of funding. Seven years ago, Brett himself was an early investor and believer in Richard and Michelle's vision. 'I'm passionate about innovating in this space, making sure good nutrition is accessible to families in the US and, hopefully, worldwide,' he says.

Kate Farms' products, which will soon include a range of new organic tube-feeding offerings, are now available in 95 per cent of US hospitals.

But this didn't happen without a fight. 'Honestly, we were kind of locked out,' says Brett. 'Hospitals could only buy synthetic formulas. Through a lot of research and hard work with doctors and consumers, we broke up that monopoly and created two categories in the healthcare system. One is the synthetic formula category and one is a plant-based organic category – both are now covered by insurance and offering better choices for families, dietitians and doctors.'

Kate Farms can be hard to come by south of the equator – something Brett promises will change – but with the global enteral formula market set to reach $US8.2 billion by 2027*, we can all expect a broader range of better nutrition options.

Consumers started this movement and, mercifully, the medical sector is finally catching up. We will not tolerate a substandard life for ourselves, our children and our families. Be it by way of commercial formula, blended food or a winning mix of both, tube-feeders are taking their health and happiness into their own hands.

Here's to a brighter future of fresh perspectives and exciting innovations in our burgeoning sector.

*Global Enteral Feeding Formulas Market by Product (Polymeric, Elemental, Disease-specific), Stage (Adults, Pediatrics), Application (Oncology, Gastroenterology, Neurology, Hypermetabolism), End User (Hospitals, LTCF, Home care) - Forecast to 2027. August 22. Accessed via researchandmarkets.com/r/xnx85g.

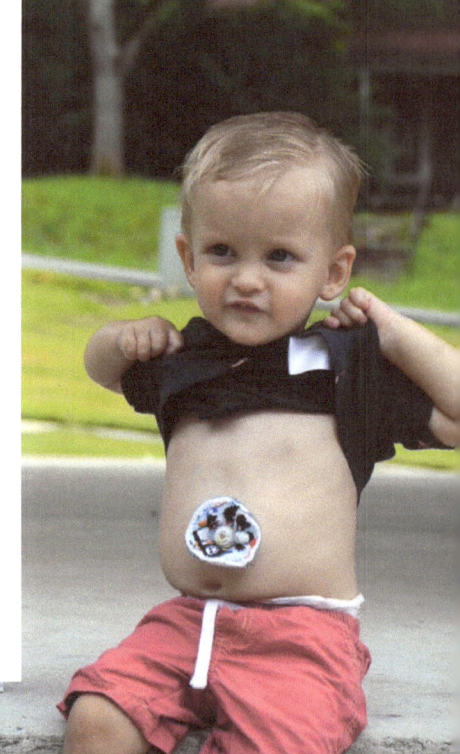

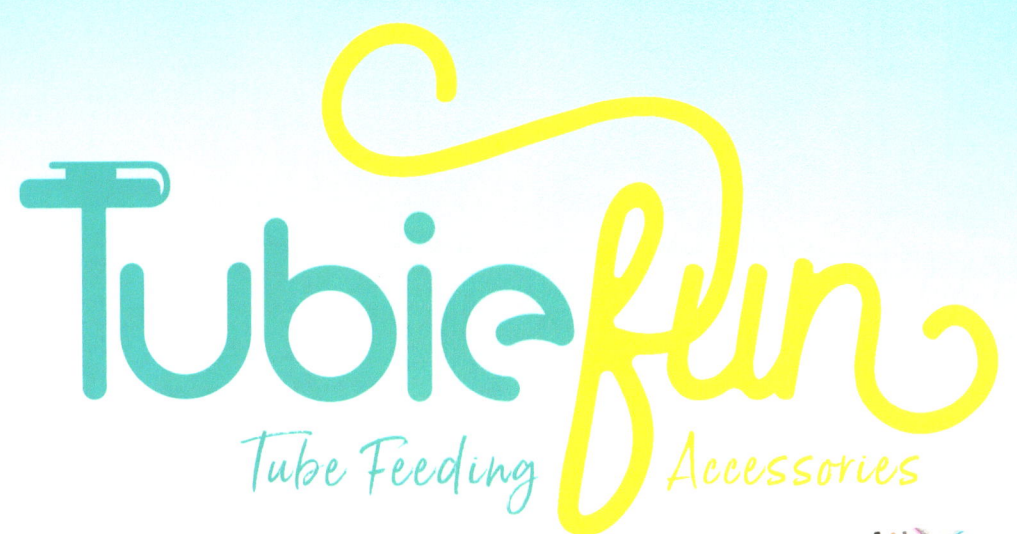

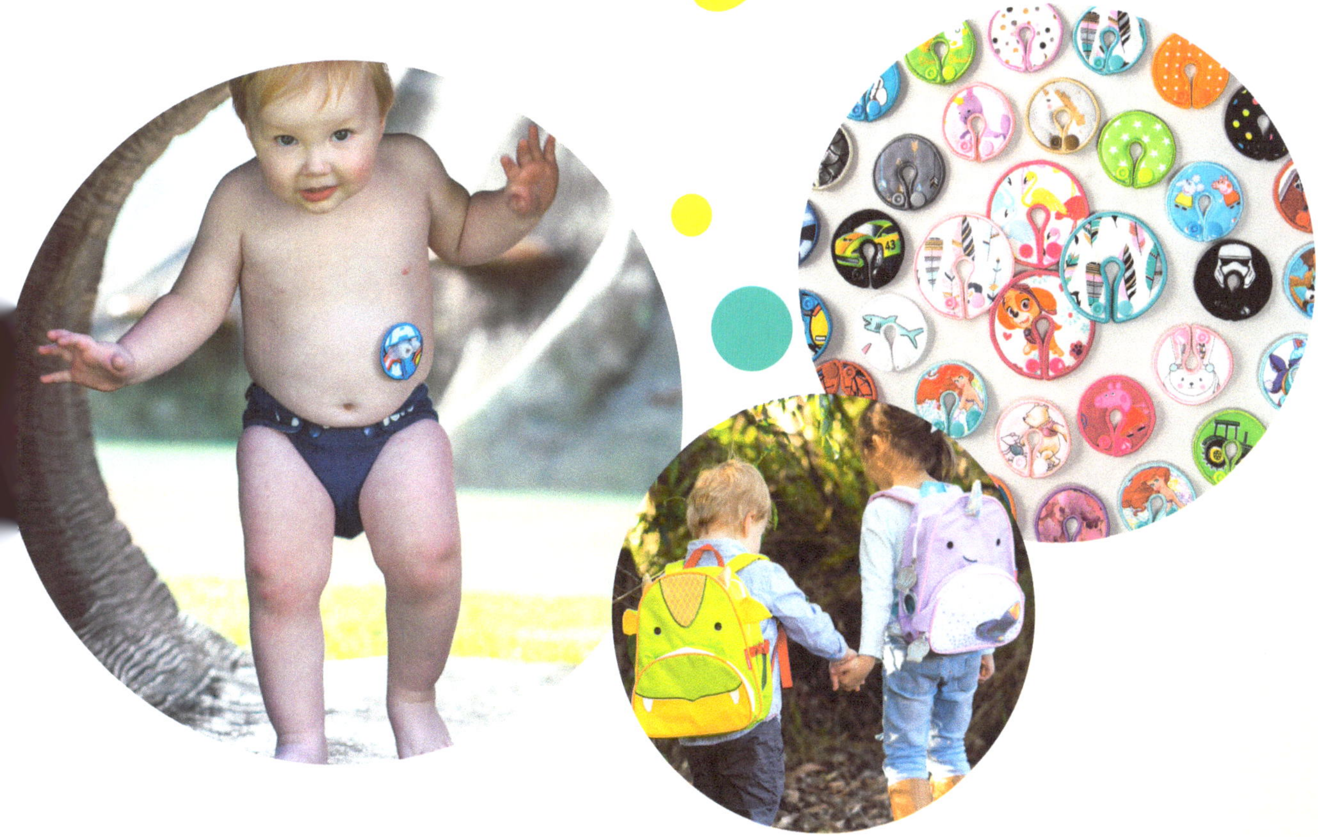

www.tubiefun.com.au

Feeding Tube Supplies & Accessories

For All Ages

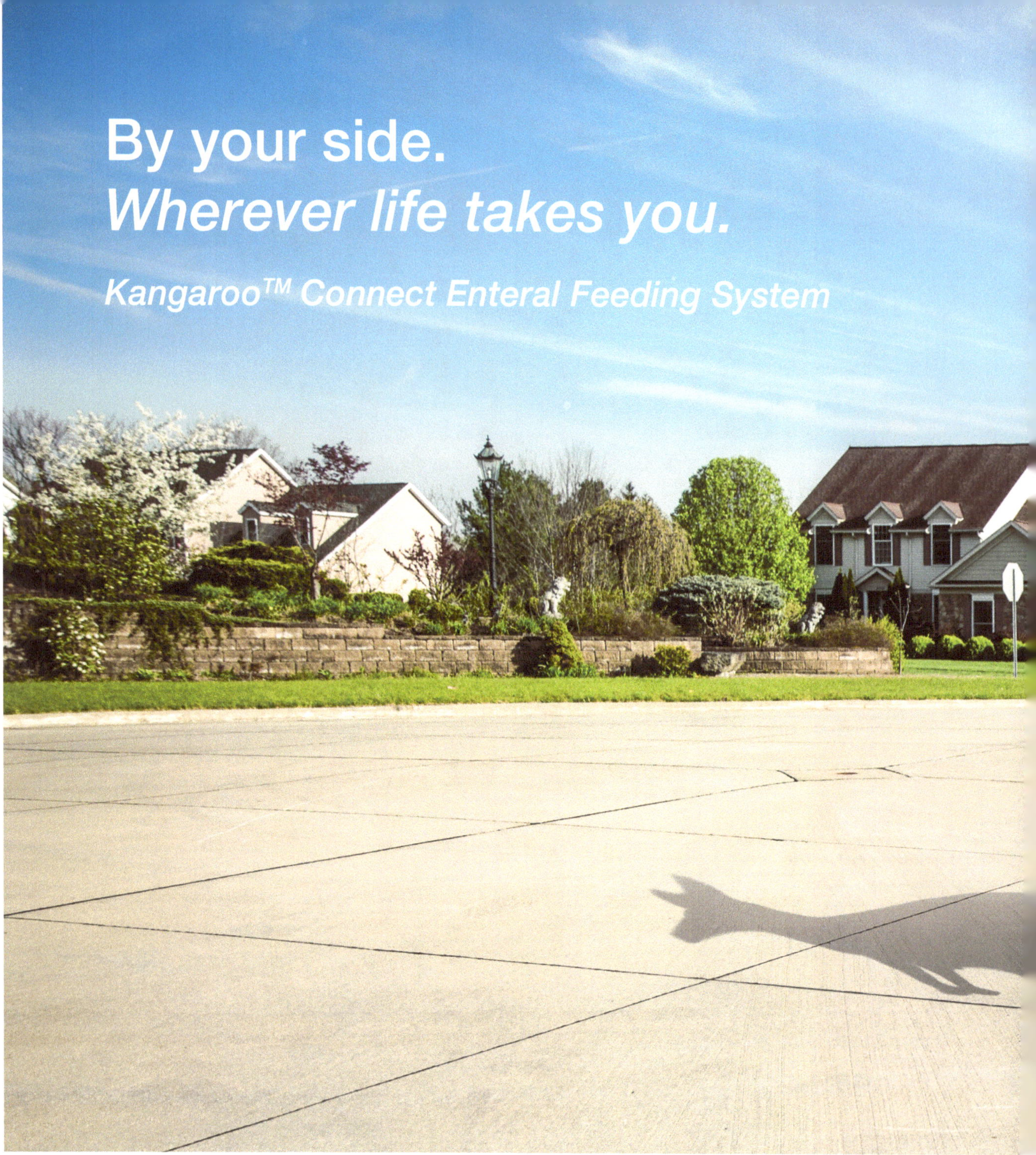

By your side.
Wherever life takes you.

Kangaroo™ Connect Enteral Feeding System

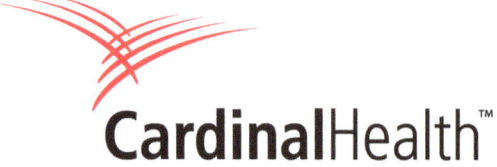

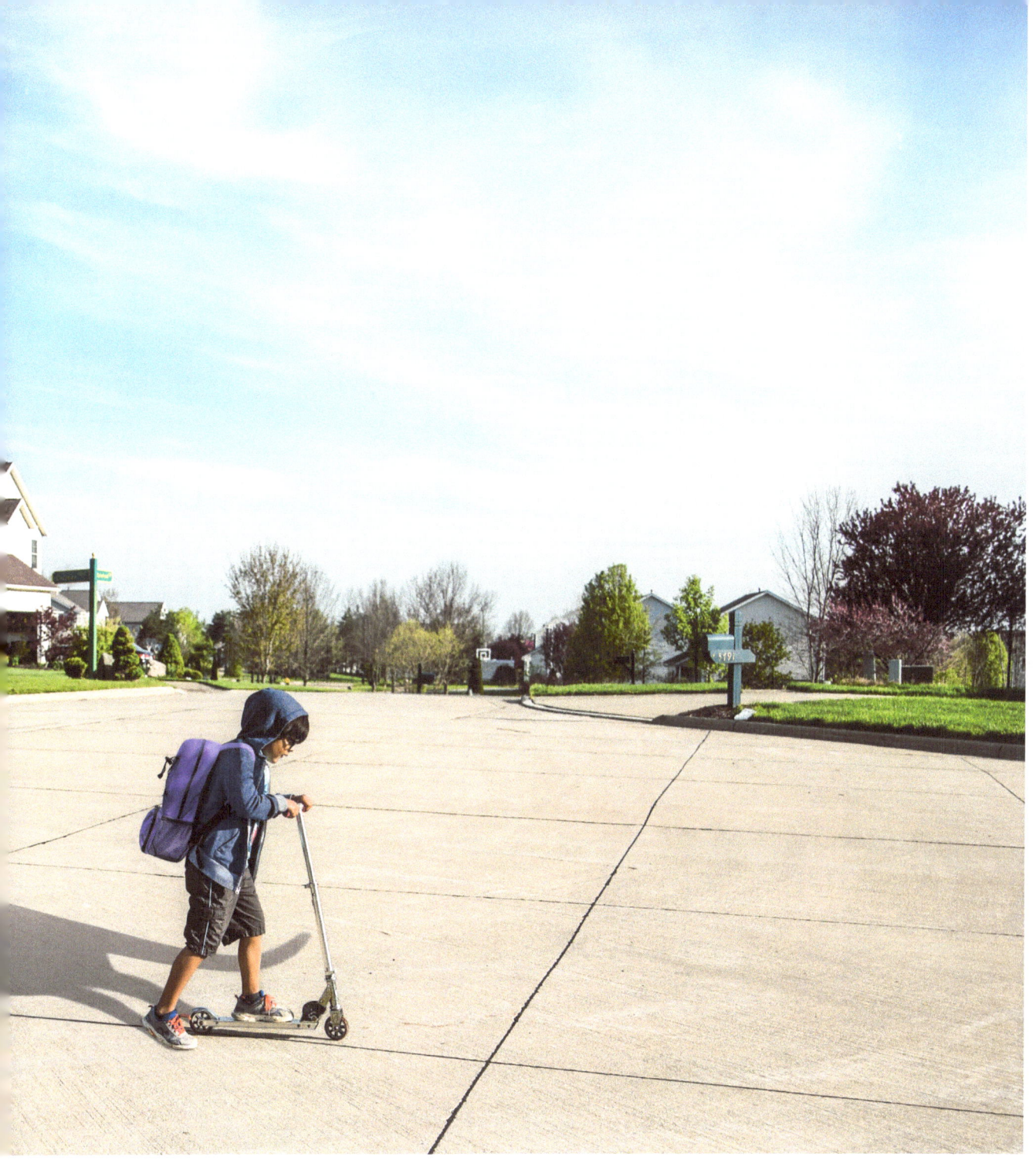

cardinalhealth.com.au/kangaroo

Cardinal Health Australia, Level 2, 5 Eden Park Drive,
North Ryde, NSW 2113 Australia

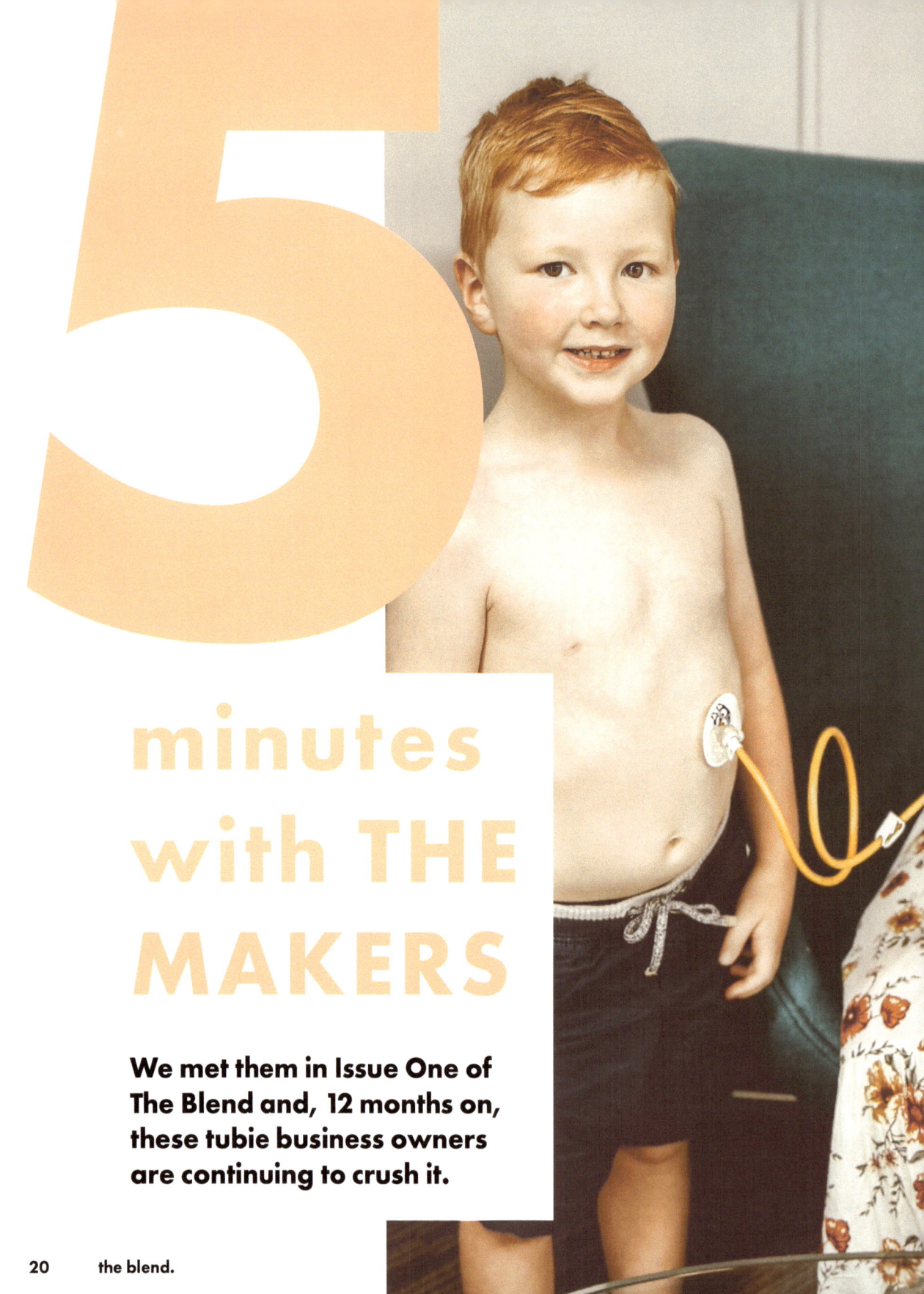

5 minutes with THE MAKERS

We met them in Issue One of The Blend and, 12 months on, these tubie business owners are continuing to crush it.

/ 5 mins

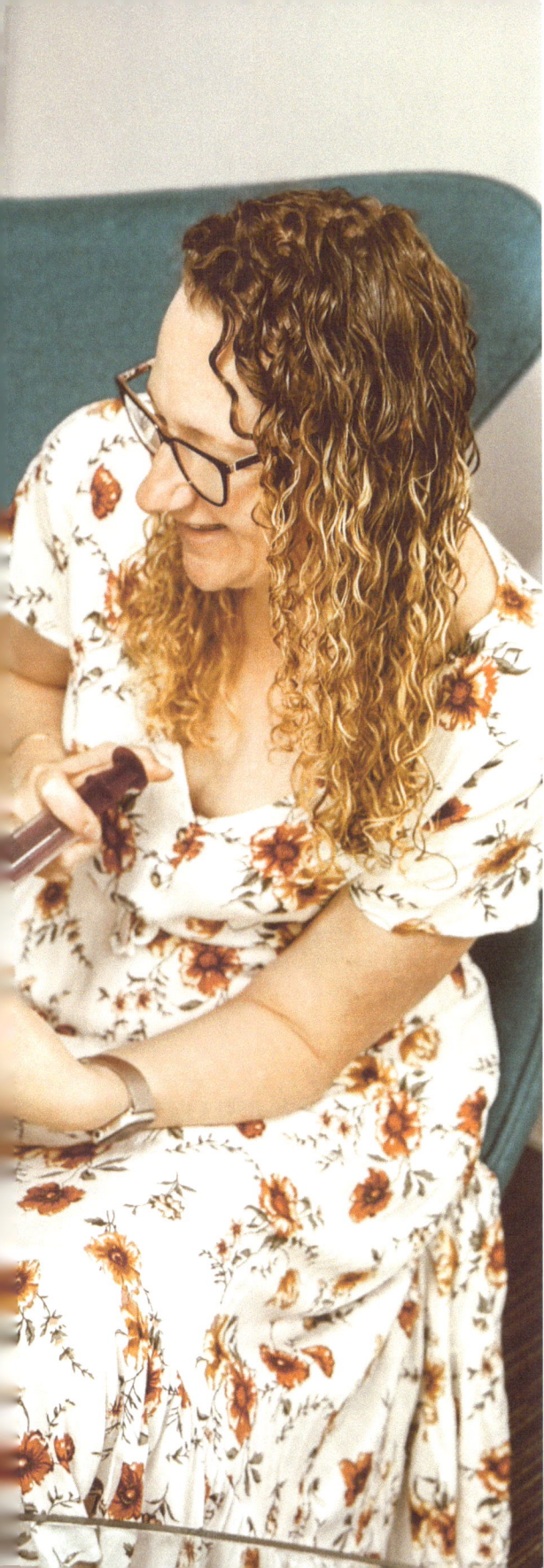

Stacey Phillips from Tubie Fun

Tubie Fun has grown immensely. We've got new staff on board – all fellow mums – to meet the demand and get our products out to more people. That's what I'm excited about – having the opportunity to reach more people and help them celebrate their individuality through tube-feeding.

I want people to love their tubes and enjoy tube-feeding, not be scared of it. It's definitely scary when you start but if our products can reduce fear, it means the world to us because we were also those scared people to begin with.

Callum, my son who tube-feeds, has been diagnosed with autism and ADHD and his oral feeding has taken a bit of a backstep, so we're taking things at his pace. Our amazing dietitian and speech therapist are working closely together to encourage him on his feeding journey – and blends have been our biggest life-saver.

Unfortunately my own health has taken a turn over the last 12 months. After years of not knowing what's going on with my body, I was diagnosed with Ehlers-Danlos syndrome. I've had to make a lot of changes so that I can still support myself and my family, but also keep our business going, because I'm not prepared to give up on my Tubie Fun dream.

We've been making personalised wheelchair covers for the Hoggi Bingo specialised stroller – and things like this really change conversations. Instead of people saying, 'why is your child in a wheelchair?' They can go, 'wow, that's really cool!'

I had a mother reach out to me who had really bad anxiety about taking her son out and everybody staring. She said: 'I'm so thankful for the wheelchair cover because it's reduced my anxiety and we can just celebrate him being out.'

Feedback like that gives me all the feels.

tubiefun.com.au

@tubiefunau

@tubiefun

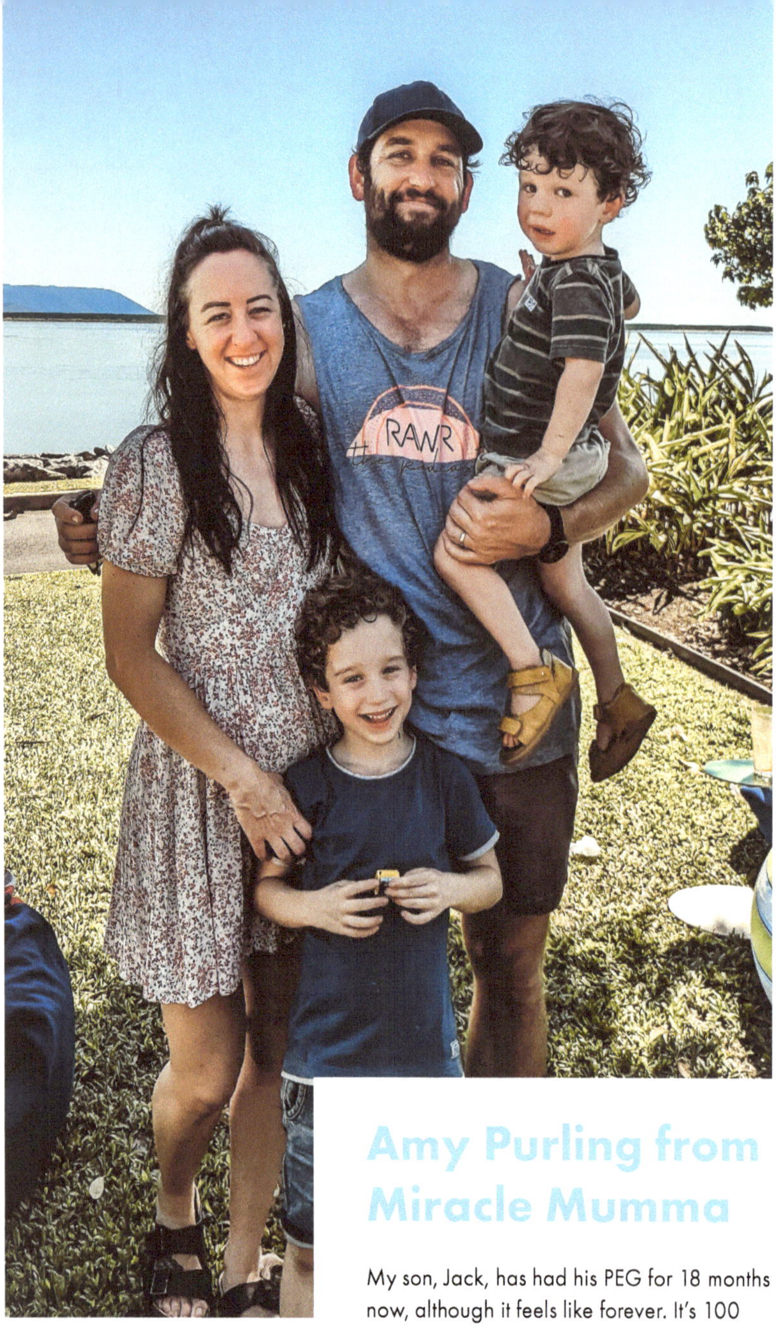

Amy Purling from Miracle Mumma

My son, Jack, has had his PEG for 18 months now, although it feels like forever. It's 100 per cent our 'normal' now and while we've had some ups and downs with infections, it's been the best thing for him. Jack calls it his 'Billy' button and he just adores pretending to tube-feed his Billy Bear which has a PEG just like him.

We've had some setbacks this winter, with a tube-wean attempt ending in a chronic wet cough that landed Jack in hospital for a two-week respiratory 'tune-up' of his lungs, marking his sixth anaesthetic in his short little life. Unfortunately the antibiotics and chest physiotherapy weren't very successful and after recurrent viral infections, he wound up on a long-term course of steroids for uncontrolled asthma. We were told once again to stop all fluids orally.

Thankfully Jack is still able to eat orally and still loving it – his favourite foods are pizza, pear and fruit purée. We have accepted that he's doing things in his own time, like he always has.

We've just moved to a new home in a small country town and the change of lifestyle has been incredible for us all. Jack and his older brother, James, spend every waking moment exploring outdoors, creating fairy gardens, riding their bikes and kicking the football. Jack is doing amazingly in all other aspects of life and is still the cheekiest, most energetic and fun little boy I know, despite all the hurdles.

In terms of Miracle Mumma, I'm excited to announce that we recently teamed up with The Travelling Tubie Project and together have launched a set of Tubie Milestone Cards that bring brightness, hope and fun to the tubie journey. The cards allow you to capture and celebrate your little one's bravery, superpowers and progress throughout their tube-feeding journey, from 'Oops! I pulled out my feeding tube' to 'I was brave for my button change' – a beautiful acknowledgement of their ability and courage no matter what challenges they face.

We also now stock The Travelling Tubie Project printed nasogastric tube tapes and I can hand-on-my-heart say there really isn't anything better than seeing photos of little ones rocking their tapes and holding their milestone cards with pride. I just love what I do and I feel truly blessed to be a part of this community.

miraclemumma.com.au

 @miraclemumma

 @miraclemumma

/ 5 mins

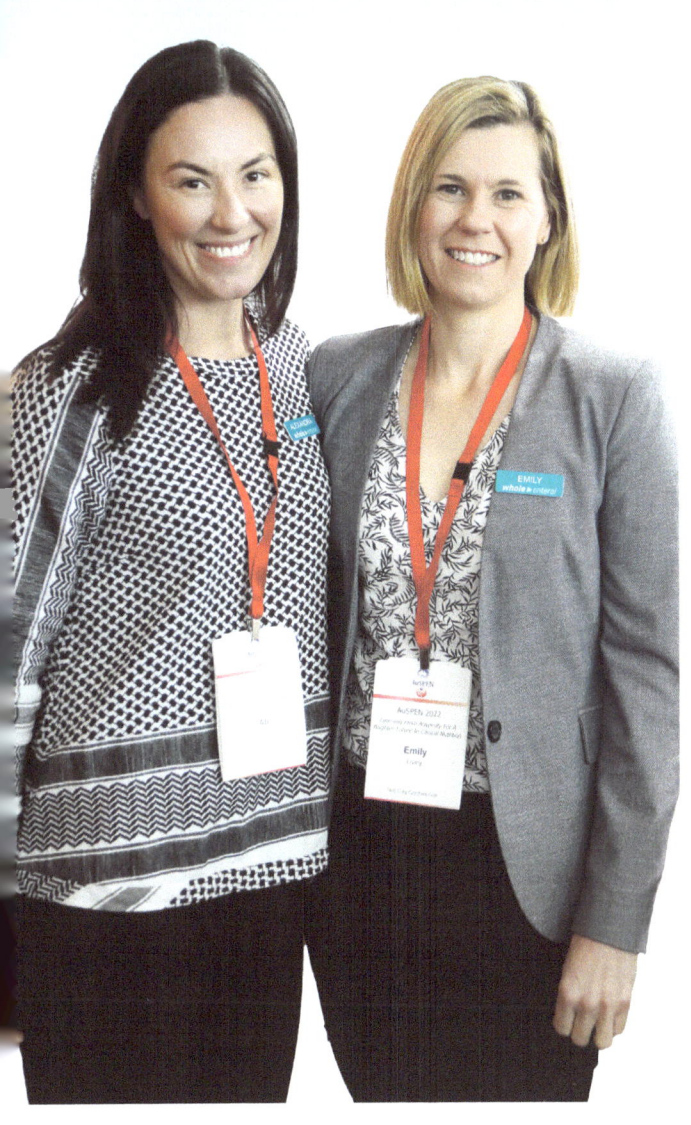

Ali Howell and Emily Lively from Whole Enteral

It's been a busy time for the team at Whole Enteral. In the past 12 months we've successfully completed our first full-scale production run, which means no more out-of-stock notices! We've also gone through a rebrand and have had a great response to the subscription products we now offer. Additionally, we've been concentrating on streamlining our NDIS invoice process. We know first-hand just how time-consuming NDIS admin can be.

One of our most valued activities has been sharing Enrich – our nutritionally formulated meal replacement – at the Dietitians Australia and AuSPEN conferences. These were fantastic opportunities to speak with clinicians all around Australia and hear their feedback and interest in our product.

We manage Whole Enteral alongside our day jobs. This means Emily has been running her feeding therapy centre, Lively Eaters, while in the final stages of completing her paediatric feeding and enteral tube weaning PhD, all while contributing to Whole Enteral in her role as co-founder.

As for me (Ali here, co-founder of Whole Enteral), the juggle is real. I'm currently working as a project manager in the finance industry while meeting the demands of life with three kids.

Kiki, my daughter who has Kabuki syndrome, continues to be a source of inspiration on the days when it all seems too much. The resilience kids with disabilities have puts me to shame – even on my best days.

What's next for us? Watch this space for exciting new product variants and the launch of our new website!

whole.net.au
@whole_en
@WHOLE.en

the blend.

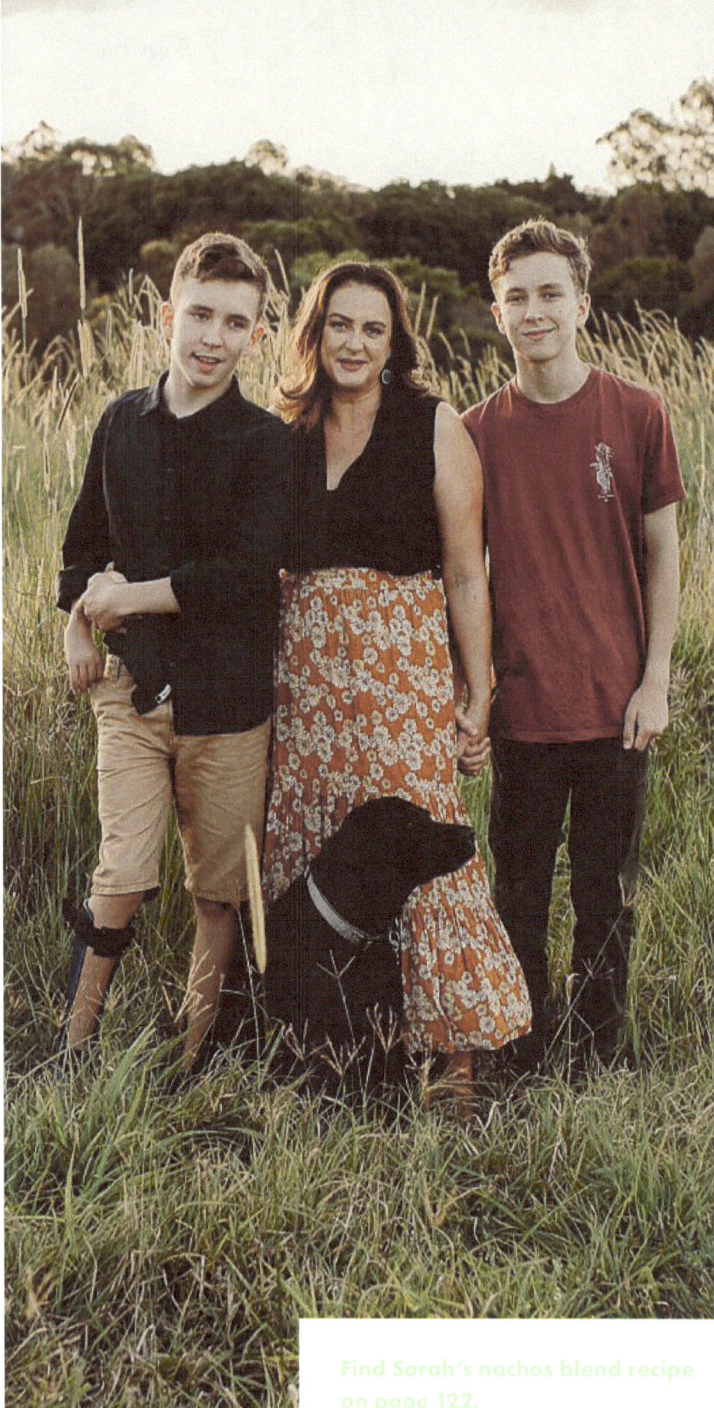

Sarah Thomas from Wholesome Blends

In the past year, the Australian tube-feeding space has grown faster than I've ever seen before. Wholesome Blends has been a big part of that growth and we continue to support families with blending at home – and also the medical community by raising awareness around the benefits of real food.

I truly believe that we all should be consuming a variety of nutrients, not just a sole source of nutrition. I don't eat the same thing every day, nor do I want my children to. And let's face it, don't we all want that occasional naughty treat? It should be no different for our tubies. My son, Lewis, loves it when he gets a dessert blend!

This past year has seen us developing more flavours in the Wholesome Blends range and employing a small in-house team. Through partnerships with local disability organisations and schools, we offer work experience for people with disabilities and students in our warehouse.

The students in these groups think we are helping them out, but I think it's the other way around. I get so much joy from young people asking me about Wholesome Blends and learning about tube-feeding.

We were excited to partner with the International Dysphagia Diet Standardisation Initiative (IDDSI) to be the first real-food enteral feed to display the IDDSI rating on our pouches. Wholesome Blends is now working closely with IDDSI to raise the bar on international standards for all enteral feeds.

On a personal level, I'm also excited to be launching in-person, one-on-one blending classes for NDIS participants and their families.

Chatting with tube-feeding families is still my favourite thing to do. I love when a family is just starting out and I can give them the confidence to blend at home.

Image: Jenna McKenzie from Terra Rosa Photography

Find Sarah's nachos blend recipe on page 122.

- wholesomeblends.com.au
- @wholesomeblendsau
- Wholesome Blends

Personal accounts.

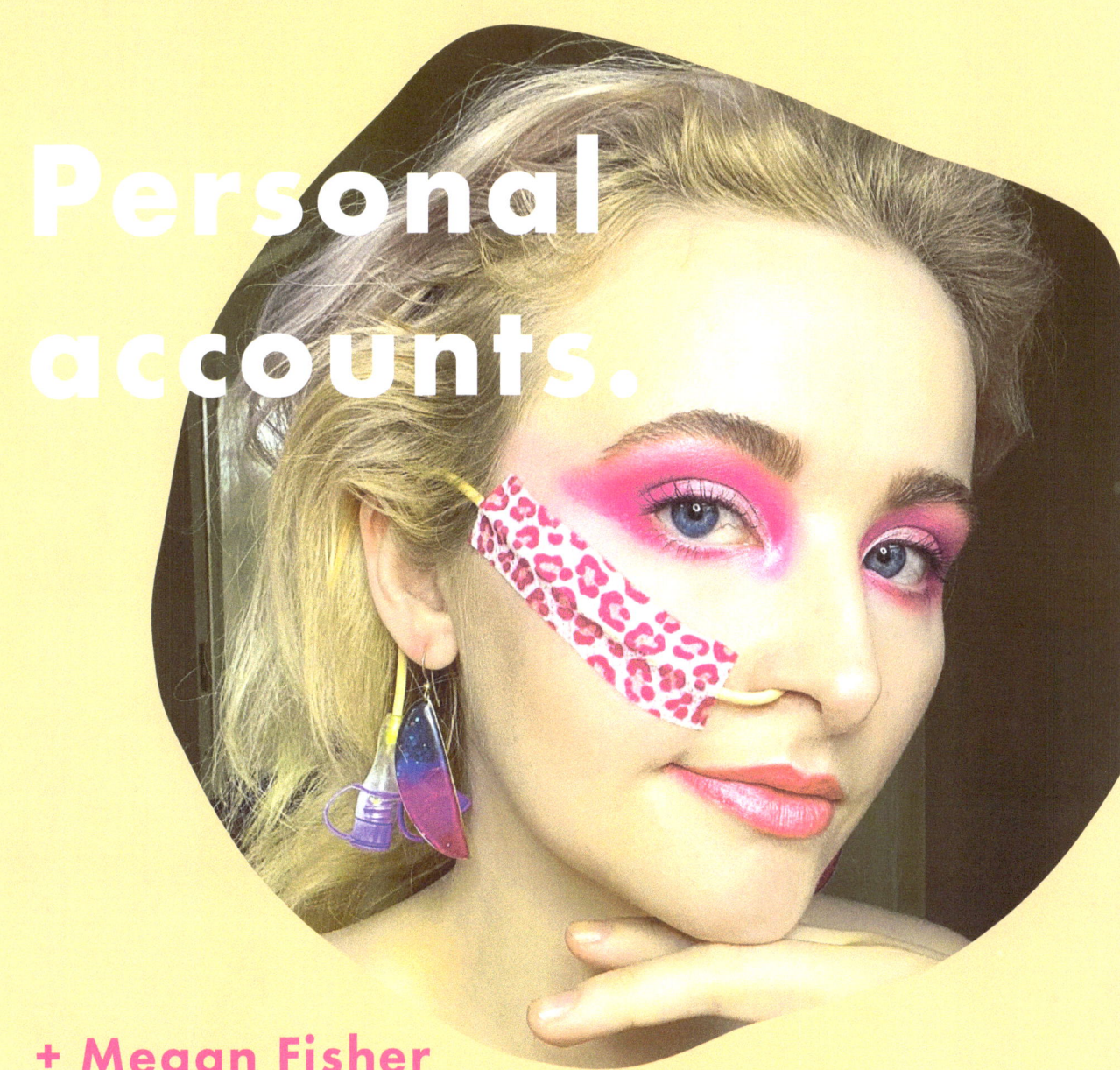

+ **Megan Fisher**
+ **Alexander Vane**
+ **Jess Cochran & Deren Kıralp**
+ **Pedro Relvas**

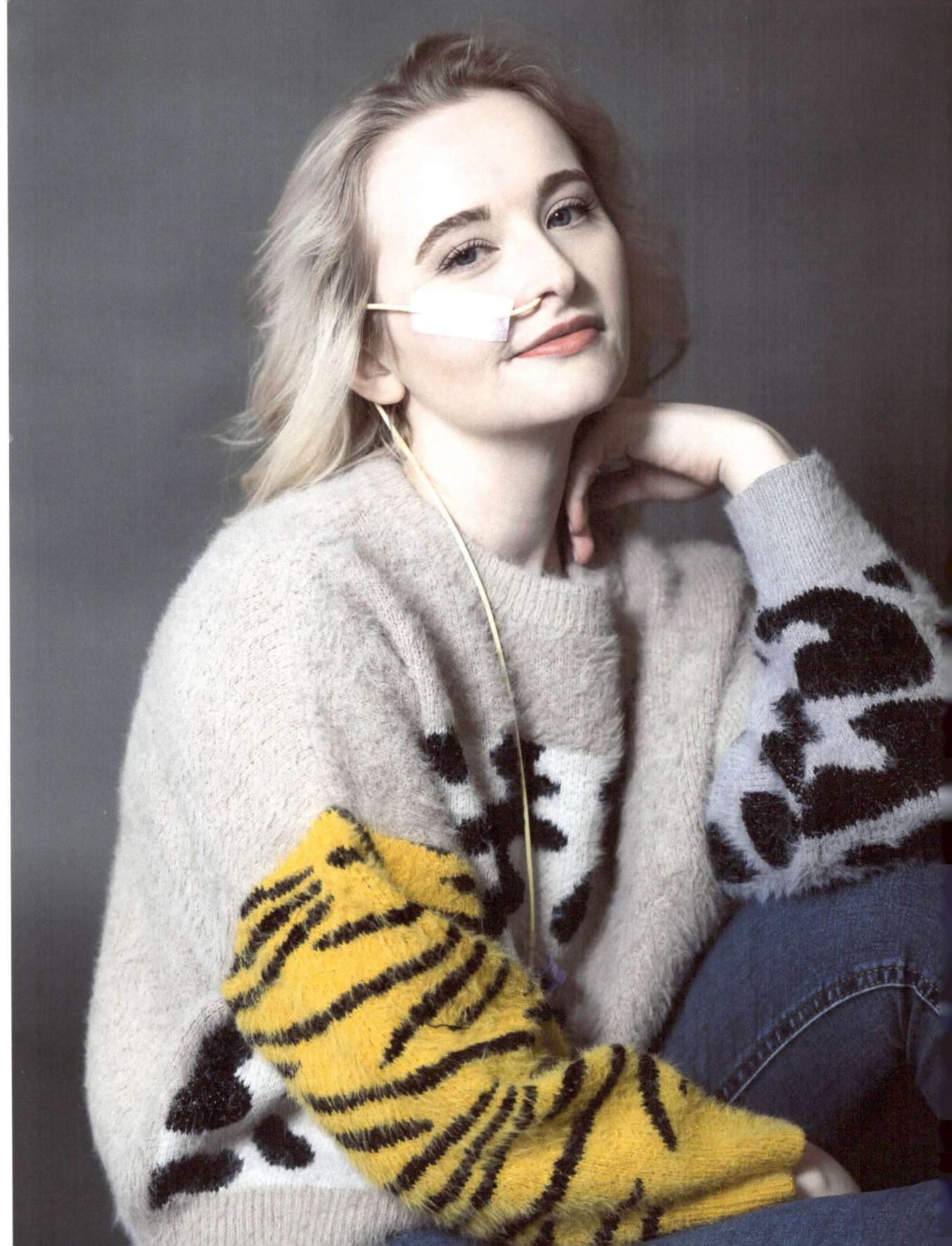

/ personal accounts

Chronically

Megan Fisher was a bodybuilder, champion equestrian and member of the British Army Reserve when, days after having her first child, she developed maternal sepsis. Since then, a landslide of conditions has dramatically impacted her body – but a new passion also emerged. Meet The Chronic Makeup Artist, a beauty influencer whose feeding tube launched her rise to fame.

You've been through so much since becoming a parent. How have you felt about not getting the 'typical' motherhood experience? I had severe sepsis two weeks after giving birth, so I had a short period of that perfect motherhood bubble. Then all of a sudden I had mastitis showing up in my breast, and three hours after getting antibiotics from my GP I was being rushed to hospital in an ambulance. For three months after that I couldn't walk, function, or do anything for myself. And then once I recovered physically, my PTSD kicked in.

The worst thing about this was that my daughter, Mollie, was my trigger. Every time she vomited – and babies vomit a lot – I'd put my hands over my head, put my head between my knees and scream. My husband Scott would run to help her, but I would just freeze. And that was the worst thing for me. My body was shutting me out of being a mother. I did therapy and my PTSD got better but even now, if she's sick, it still triggers me.

I dreamt of teaching my daughter to ride horses, because I rode horses from age two. I can't even sit on a horse right now – I'm currently using a wheelchair – but I'm always there for Mollie. Even when I'm in hospital, Scott will Skype me and she'll talk to me.

Motherhood is not the way I wanted it to be but I know many people don't get a chance at it, so I'm taking all I can get from this. I've spoken to other mothers with chronic illness who are tube-feeding and we pick each other up. I have one friend that says: 'You're still her mother. That girl looks up to you and loves you, regardless of what shape you're in.' >>

creative

the blend.

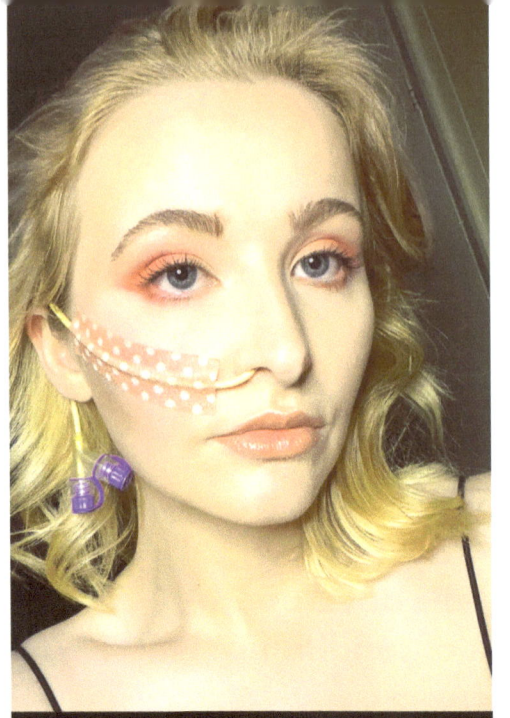

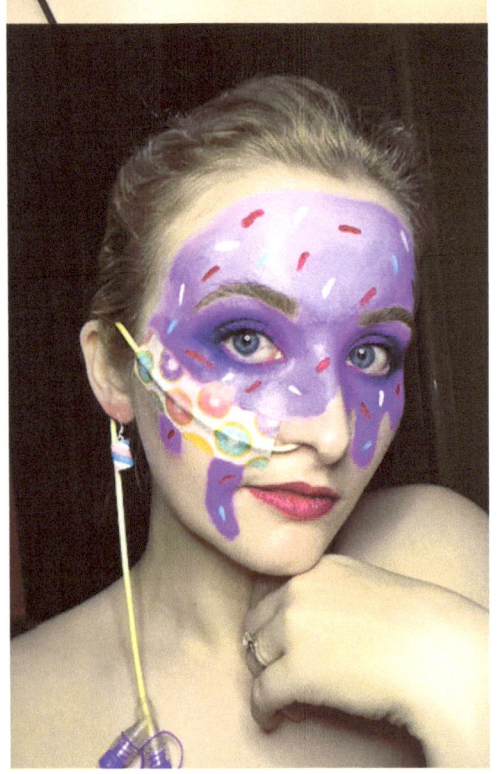

I'll bet Mollie takes all of the medical stuff in her stride. It's just so normal for her, she doesn't question it. The other day, when she saw another woman in a wheelchair, she didn't say, 'why is she in a wheelchair?' she said, 'Mummy, she's got a red wheelchair! You've got an orange one'.

She doesn't focus on the negatives. For her – and kids like her, who grow up around long-term disability – all the taboo and the panic around seeing a disabled person is stripped away.

At Christmas, Mollie's first instinct was to ask Santa for a Barbie doll in a wheelchair, because it looked like her – that's why I'm in a wheelchair. I can't walk and am currently doing rehab. For me, going from having legs to not having legs is just unbearable.

Before I got sick I was weightlifting and riding horses. I have a degree in sports science. I was working in the army and wanted to become a physiotherapist, but all of that went straight out the window. So it was a question of, what can I physically do now that I enjoy?

Holding a round makeup brush can be quite hard – my grip goes from my right hand – so I use Kohl Kreatives brushes that are squared off and designed for

> "She clearly sees me, even though I feel invisible to her. She sees me as a good person, not this person tangled up in leads."

mummy. That was the point for me where I realised, I am a mother. She clearly sees me, even though I feel invisible to her. She sees me as a good person, not this person tangled up in leads.

That idea of being invisible – in a broader, societal sense – is something you push against with your makeup artistry. Tell me how you came to start honing this skill in the midst of your health struggles. It began in November 2021, when my mental health plummeted. In September I'd had a suspected stroke which affected the right side of my body people with fine-motor limitations.

I started off sticking to just my eyes, whereas now I do a full face and often quirky looks.

I'm not a professional in any shape or form. The other day I was looking at one of my videos, turning to Scott and saying, 'my line work is horrendous'. And Scott was like, 'at least you're doing something'.

Makeup is my outlet. The colours I use really resonate with how I'm feeling. If I do pink and sparkly, that's a good day. Other days I might use dark or more emotive colours. You might have seen my ABC look? >>

/ personal accounts

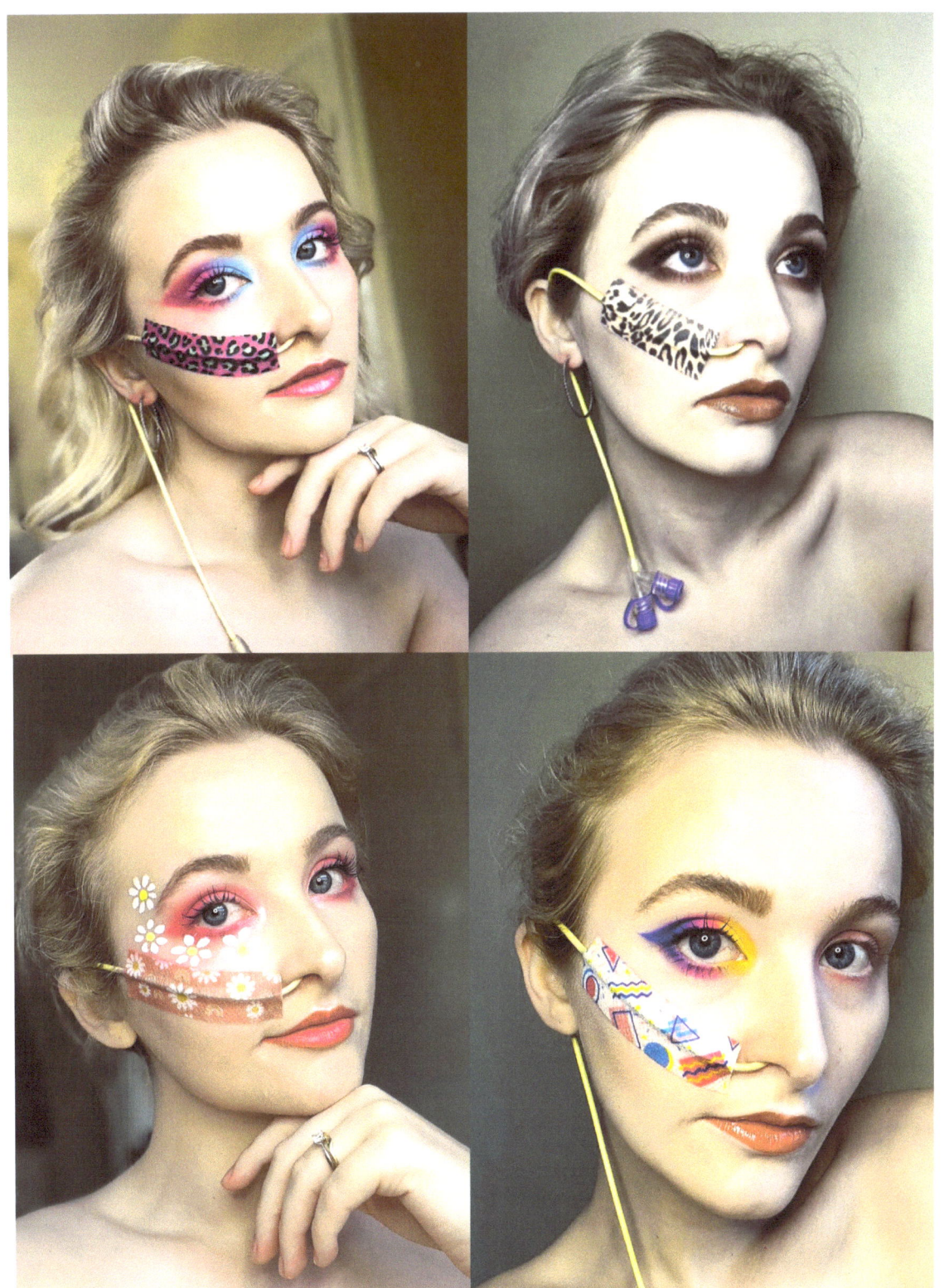

the blend.

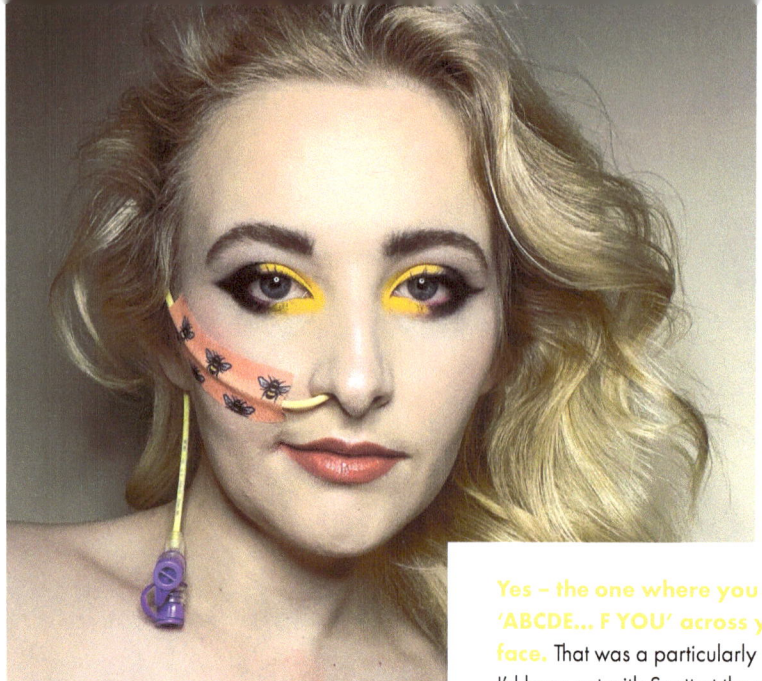

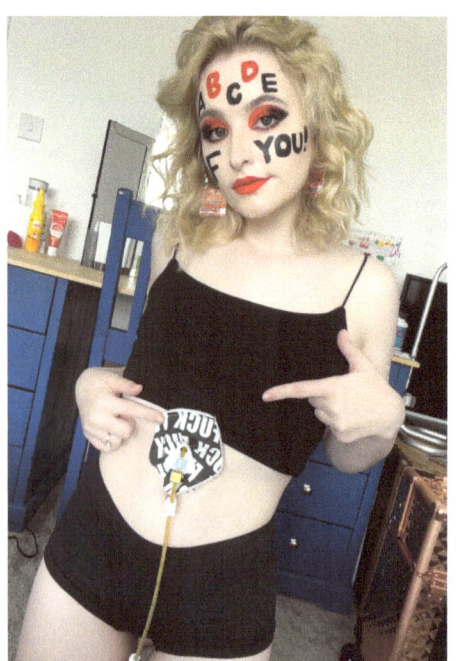

Yes – the one where you painted 'ABCDE... F YOU' across your face. That was a particularly bad day. I'd been out with Scott at the pub. The whole place was rammed and yet no one would sit at the table beside us. Five or six couples walked up, looked at me in my wheelchair with my tube and then turned around, walked away and stood.

While I was getting more and more self-conscious, Scott got to the point where, when the next couple came up to us and were about to retreat, he said: 'Just sit down. We're not going to bite. There's nothing disgusting about this. You can eat through your mouth, some people have to eat differently.'

Well said, Scott. And on that note, tell me, when did you start eating differently? The sepsis happened after I gave birth and as the months went by, gastrointestinal and neurological symptoms started appearing and kept progressing. In January 2021, it was like my body just gave up.

Over the next six months I lost over 25kg because I was vomiting everything I ate and drank. I also had repeated anaphylaxis and swelling. Eventually I was diagnosed with epilepsy and mast cell activation syndrome (MCAS). Essentially, I'm allergic to all food. That's why my body was getting rid of it.

It got to the point where my weight was getting dangerously low, so I got a nasogastric (NG) tube, but once we worked out my stomach couldn't tolerate food, I switched to a nasojejunal (NJ) tube. However, when I'd have seizures – and I have tonic-clonic, or grand mal seizures – the NJ would flip out of my intestine and into my stomach.

In the space of six months I had 10 NJs. I'd get a tube placed, seize, and be back in the next day getting it replaced again.

That must have been incredibly traumatic. Yes. And it meant I lost more weight. I got admitted to hospital because I was going downhill and the doctors diagnosed me with gastroparesis and decided that the NJ was doing me more trauma than good, so we went to a gastrostomy-jejunostomy (G-J) tube. In the months since that's gone in I've had several major infections, so more tests are being run to get to the bottom of that.

If you're allergic to food, what goes into your tube? This has been a journey as well. After a lot of trial and error I'm now on a semi broken-down food. It's not great – I still have reactions – but I'm getting nutrition in. Orally, I can have potatoes, gluten-free bread and a small amount of tuna and egg, and I've been trialling medications to help me eat more, because I'd love to go down the blended-diet route.

Usually I'm on 24/7 feeds, but today I'm not hooked up because I'm waiting on my medication delivery – the drugs to keep me stable enough to accept my feed. I've just been running fluids – but that's a bad day for me.

/ **personal accounts**

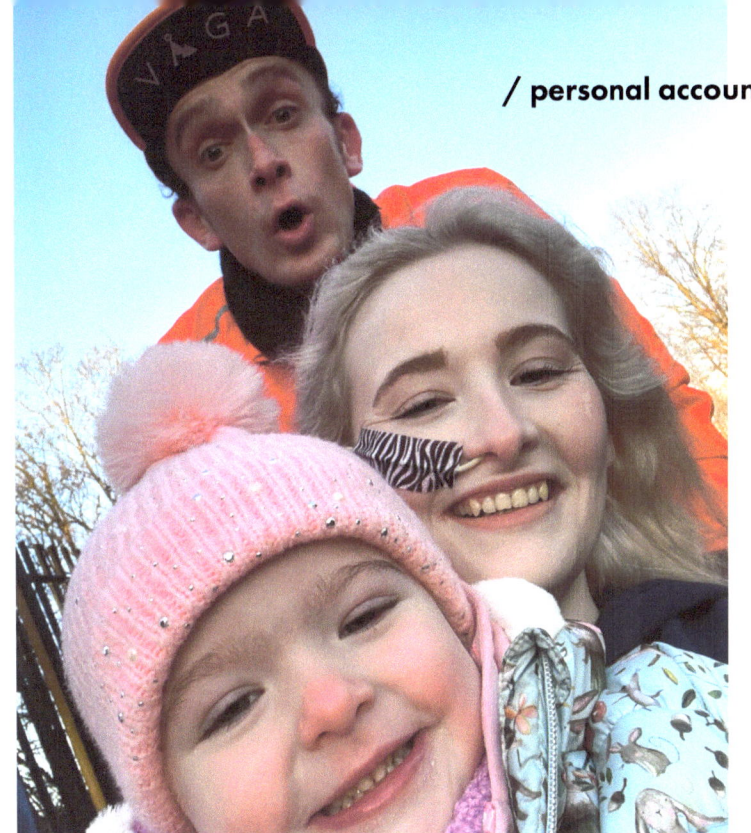

Speaking of your medication, Scott made news headlines when he completed 27 marathons in 27 days to help fund research into MCAS. This epic effort was inspired by the 27 different medications you need to take every day – is it still this many? I'm now on 30-plus meds and Scott's already planning his next great mission to raise money for MCAS. He's my rock. Scott has stood by me every single step of the way and I'm very, very fortunate. I have friends in the tube-feeding community who've had people just turn on them, saying it's their fault. It's not anyone's fault if they're struggling to eat. It's not like we can just click our fingers and eat a chicken dinner.

Scott is a massive advocate for my makeup work, too. He's faithfully sat through every episode of Glow Up and keeps coaxing me to apply. Sophie Baverstock, who won season three, has autism – and Scott says, if Sophie can do it, why can't you? They haven't yet had physical disability represented on there – certainly no one in a wheelchair.

Please do apply for Glow Up – a wildly popular TV show that crowns 'Britain's next makeup star', for readers who aren't familiar. You say you're not a professional makeup artist and yet you've already nabbed gigs in the industry. What does this look like? I work with small brands and help promote them – and now I'm working with About-Face beauty by [American singer-songwriter] Halsey. That was the major win for me, not only because it's a huge brand in the industry, but also because Halsey has MCAS and Ehlers-Danlos syndrome, which I have as well. Her products don't react with me because she formulates them without nasties.

> "Your limitations are not limitations – they are giving you life and a purpose."

A lot of makeup does cause allergic reactions for me, but I keep working with my EpiPen beside me. I know people must think, why the hell are you doing that to yourself? But I'd rather be doing my makeup, having a reaction, taking my emergency meds, cracking on and just having that positive thing in my life. I'll regret it a couple of hours later, but in the moment, it's all I want to do. I'm holding on to it, no matter what my body is trying to tell me.

It's worth it – and it's what works for you. What advice do you have for people who are new to tube-feeding? Just stay open. Talk to everyone in the community. Don't shut yourself off because once you shut yourself off – and I've done it myself – your mental health crumbles. And no matter how many medical professionals say you won't be able to do this and you won't be able to do that, find a way. Your limitations are not limitations – they are giving you life and a purpose. Don't give up, just keep going.

 @chronicmakeupartist

the blend. 31

Acquired taste

With a chronic inflammatory condition and lengthy list of allergies, 18-year-old Alexander Vane has lived on commercial formula through a G-tube since he was seven. However, a new medication has this New Zealander feasting on a delicious array of foods for the first time.

/ **personal accounts**

What's it like going to school with a gastrostomy (G) tube? When I played hockey or soccer we'd put this big band around my body and stuff it with cotton wool to protect my tube – that was quite noticeable. But during school it hasn't been a big deal because I've always had great friends there to support me.

I'd have most of my feeds in a separate room during morning tea or lunch, but they'd join me for that and we'd have a chat.

I'm already sensing that for my young son, Arlo, tube-feeds at school are not an issue. His classmates are actually pretty interested in it. So what do you have through your tube? It's a hypoallergenic formula at the moment. I've got eosinophilic esophagitis (EoE) and I've never been able to eat enough food safely, so this formula is how I've stayed alive and continued to thrive.

Do you eat anything orally? In the last two years we've come across a miracle drug, which our government funding agency eventually approved after saying I 'wasn't exceptional enough' a few times. Since we got approval I've been injecting it once a week and we've been able to slowly introduce foods. So I've actually got a bit of a diet now, which is incredible.

I've always loved cooking. Before I could eat I'd just put rubber gloves on and try to help out where I could. So I've always been interested in food and being able to eat it now is a really interesting learning curve. Chip sandwiches, for example. Kids love them when they're small but I missed all of that. So I'm coming across them now and telling all my friends, 'oh my gosh, have you tried this? This is amazing!' and they're like, 'yeah, maybe when I was like six'.

I'd argue chip sandwiches are amazing at any age. How does it feel to be eating food now, after years of nothing? Before the miracle drug I was able to have a few fruits and vegetables – it was about eight in total. But even they ended up being unsafe, so it was back to no food. I've eaten a little bit over the years, but nowadays, coming across different types of meats, breads, firm things, soft things, is really interesting. And all the different flavours as well, which is great.

It must be mind-blowing – I've caught you at a very interesting time. Prior to that, when you were in social situations centred around food, was that hard? I definitely struggled with it, especially at times like Christmas. Growing up with my tube made me realise how much society revolves around food and I definitely felt like I was missing out.

But I tried to involve myself where I could, and Mum and Dad always made an effort. There are so many different ways you can cook a potato or apple, so we would try and work them into celebratory meals.

How did you explain the way you eat when meeting new people? I think my go-to line was probably something like, my body rejects the food that I eat, so I substitute it for a drink that has all the vitamins and nutrients I need to keep me going. My high-school years are when I've had to explain it the most. But I've kept a really solid friendship group all the way through and they all have their own little ways of explaining it.

How are they feeling about your new-found diet? After a year of being on this miracle drug, my mates and I got dressed up in suits, went bowling and then went back to one of their houses and cooked a meal together. This was a really big step for me because that was the first time I'd ever had food that was cooked outside of my own home. We all sat around in our suits with identical meals of potatoes, steak and salads, and celebrated.

That's a very cool story... It's the little things like that that make everything so much easier to deal with. That's a memory I'll have forever. I won't always remember the nights my pump alarms were going off, or when my feed leaked and I had to have a shower at four in the morning. But I'll remember the really good stuff. That's what has got me through the last 10 years of having a tube. >>

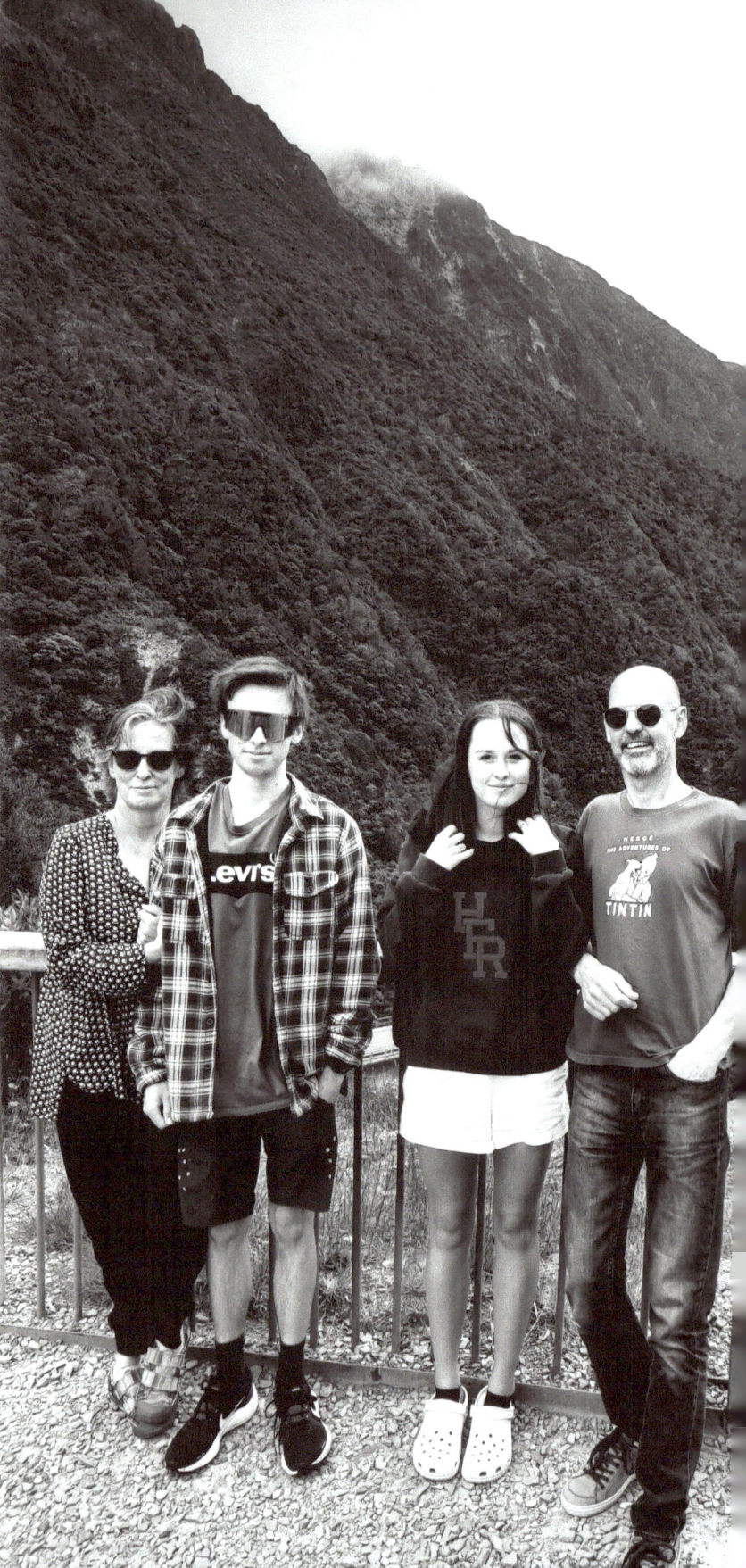

Do you get into the G-tube accessories? Arlo has some very cute button pads, but that might be something you grow out of. I do have some and I used them quite a bit with my old tube site location to help the leaking, because that was nasty. Now I just leave it alone and clean it at night. It was something that I definitely used to worry about, because it stunk a lot. But now I just put a bunch of deodorant on and call it a day.

On the topic of potentially embarrassing odours, has tube-feeding been an issue when it comes to dating? No, not really. Most people have been really good about it and because I tend to meet people through friends, they already know what's going on. I am pretty good at being able to read someone's reaction and know who's approachable or not. It hasn't been an issue.

What advice do you have for young people who are new to tube-feeding? People are never asking about your tube to tease or be rude. Everyone has great intentions but some people might come across a bit rough or blunt. I promise you they are just curious and interested – we all want to learn. And if we're open about what we're doing, then they see a new part of the world. They see a new part of how people's lives are and become more aware of people's day-to-day challenges. And that can help them in their own life, as well.

/ **personal accounts**

Some words of wisdom from Alexander's mum, Sarah Vane

Alexander is an outlier for his condition and resistant to all treatment options, so that's how we ended up on this trial and a very new FDA [Food and Drug Administration] approved drug. Each week he has an injection that allows him to eat. Without it, he can't have any food.

We had quite the battle to get there. I'd rung all over the world – manufacturers, distributors and researchers – because we simply couldn't keep him going on amino-acid formula alone.

After being on a nasogastric (NG) tube in the neonatal intensive care unit, then drinking formula for about a year, Alexander was finally diagnosed with EoE at 15 months old, with reactions to both food and environmental triggers. He got an NG at seven years old, then switched to G-tube at eight, with a tube resiting at 15.

We had just lost our home in the 2011 Christchurch earthquake when Alexander started on his G-tube. We moved six times in three years, twice with only carry bags. Finding suitable places to live was tough when competing with so many hundreds of others.

Since then we've trialled foods off and on, then off again until 2020, when we started reintroducing food with the new medication. Don't get me started on food diaries – I have folders full of them.

Throughout all of this, Alexander has played sports. He loves going mountain biking and on an annual hike with his dad, my husband Paul. Alexander and his younger sister, Isabel, have the usual sibling rivalries but also a wonderfully tight bond. Appreciating he was missing out, she decided to give up some treat

> **"If you aren't sure, ask. And if you still aren't sure, keep asking."**

foods to show her support for him when they were younger. She has gained an understanding, responsible and caring nature that she takes out into the world.

Each age and stage has come with new challenges and I was unable to return to paid work with so much uncertainty. I spent two years going into Alexander's school to help him tube-feed until we learned there was funding for a teacher's aide. Paul went on the school camps so Alexander could take part there, too.

Being involved with school made a real difference and we could add some fun – like, 'everyone eats like Alexander for a day', or 'al-fresco' tube-feeding on sunny days on the lawn.

Sarah Gray and her organisation, ausEE Inc., have been a great source of support and information for our family. Closer to home, I joined a national clinical reference group to help improve paediatric tube-feeding in New Zealand. This group was created as a result of a directive from the health ministry in response to a patient petition – power to the people!

I was the only consumer representative alongside paediatricians, dietitians, psychologists, occupational therapists and outreach nurses – a great team who are now finally publishing, presenting and promoting a way forward.

As part of my work with this group, I designed a survey and reached out to many families who are tube-feeding. Their input was generous and so powerful. It unearthed key themes like the need for timely information, treatment, multidisciplinary support and more understanding of the emotional impact of tube-feeding. One piece of advice that rang out loud and clear was: 'If you aren't sure, ask. And if you still aren't sure, keep asking.'

When we all share, we gain company and strength beyond geographical boundaries. We make it that little bit better for others and create positive change.

 You can find some of Sarah's work, resources and support for tube-feeding at kidshealth.org.nz

Tubie to be

Journalist Kate Thomas will soon have a feeding tube placed. In an effort to face her fears around this looming unknown, she interviewed two people who are tube-feeding and making it their own. Here's where Kate's curiosity led her.

I've known for some time that tube-feeding would be a likely outcome for me. That one day I'd probably need to have my Sunday roasts blended and pumped through to my stomach. But I was harshly reminded of this likelihood early last year, when I choked on a piece of pasta.

It was my favourite meal – and pasta-bly the worst kind of reminder (forgive the pun).

Searching health advice on Google is usually considered a very bad idea. An inquisitive search about your medical condition or symptom can lead to a litany of doomsday reading – and when you search for a degenerative condition, such as mine, you may as well pack up your laptop and live today as if it's your last.

So when it came time to research tube-feeding, I was wary. I turned to Google and whispered into its search engine my questions and fears: Is tube-feeding painful? Do you leave the tube in? What specialist do you speak to about tube-feeding? Does tube-feeding limit your life?

I wanted to be prepared and know my options when meeting with a doctor. But what I found online was not what I needed or wanted to know. I was looking for something more tangible and real. I wanted the lived experiences. The funny stories of tube formula exploding all over the ceiling. The times of hopelessness, the trial and error of finding the right tube.

This was why, when approached to write this piece, I leapt at the opportunity. Here was my chance to talk to people about their experiences without feeling intrusive or nosey. I could come at this under the guise of being a journalist on the hunt for a good story, all the while inserting my personal anxieties into the interview questions.

As it turned out, this soon-to-be tubie newbie needn't have worried. All of my hesitations were about to be absolved by two conversations.

'I'm known for my obsession with bubble tea, that's my thing,' Jess Cochran says over a Zoom call.

Jess, who has a PEG-J (gastrostomy-jejunostomy) tube, is a self-declared foodie. 'Down to the bone,' she says. 'Especially being in Melbourne, we obviously have a great food scene.'

Trying to hide my shock and cautious excitement, I replied that I thought once you have a tube, you, well, can't eat food.

'No, [for me] it's encouraged,' she explains. >>

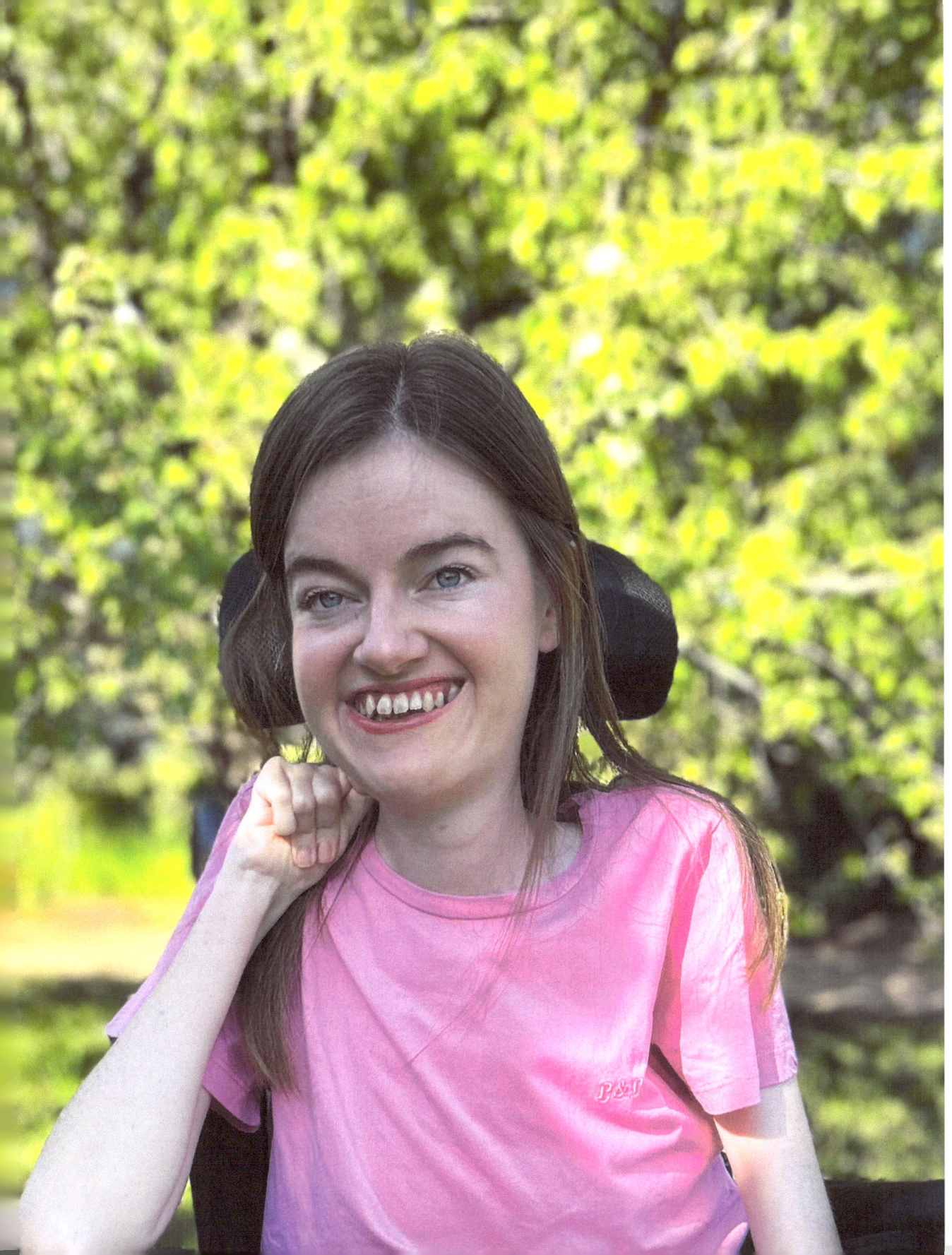

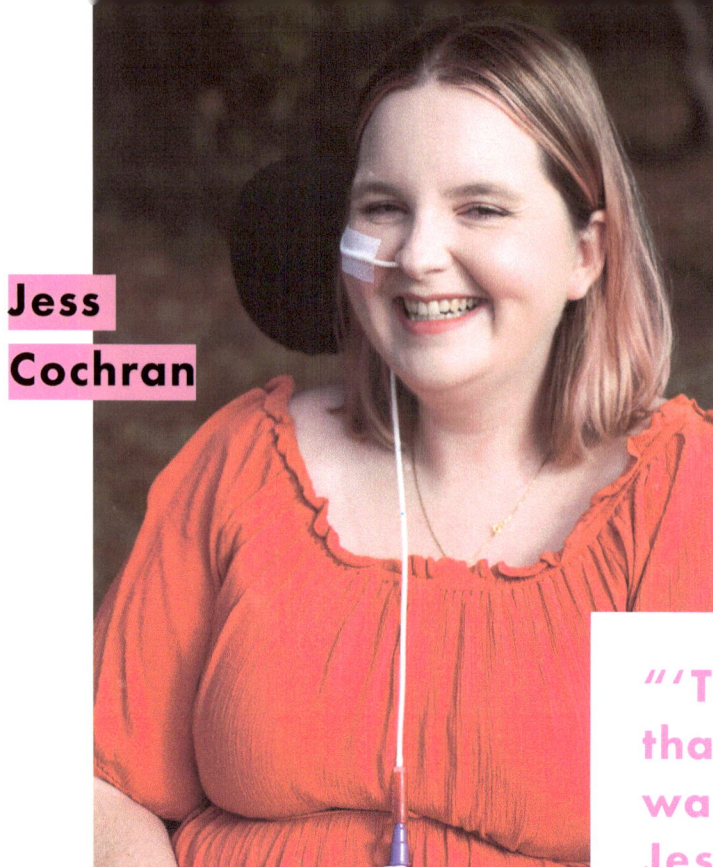

Jess Cochran

Another person who has wielded the power of social media is Deren Kıralp, who goes by the handle @whos_deren. In many respects, Deren is an ordinary 18-year-old. He loves going to the beach with friends and lives in Cyprus with his parents and twin sister. Unlike other 18-year-olds, though, he has amassed almost 165,000 followers on video-sharing app, TikTok.

'I started [making TikTok videos] in lockdown for Covid,' says Deren when we speak. 'It started as doing fun stuff

> **"'There are a lot of things that I didn't know as I was preparing myself,' Jess explains. 'So I think if you get a warning sign, start early.'"**

'In a medical way it helps you keep that muscle motility in your oesophagus. Some people may not necessarily be able to swallow food but they're still able to taste it, and chew it, then they just spit it out. As long as it's actually safe to have something in your mouth, keeping that connection is really important.'

This was one of many myths Jess would bust for me.

With wide-eyed warmth, Jess openly described her first encounters with tube-feeding and the many mishaps and challenges she experienced. She advised me to start my research early. She also emphasised the importance of finding activities that don't solely revolve around food – but to remain engaged during meal times. She said I should find a doctor who's receptive to me, but also spoke of the value of having a friend or family member as an ally at medical appointments.

'There are a lot of things that I didn't know as I was preparing myself,' Jess explains. 'So I think if you get a warning sign, start early.'

Jess's most surprising advice was to turn to social media. As part of starting to prepare for her tube-feeding journey, Jess found the online tubie community.

'It can be really hard to connect with a complete group of strangers online,' Jess says. 'But when it comes to the tubie community – whether it's an adult who's tube-fed, a parent whose children are tube-fed, or anything in between – everyone and anyone is on there. You'll reach out looking for something, or be caught on holiday when you lose your feed, and people will run to your aid. They're really such kind, incredible people.'

with my sister at home – like dances – but I deleted the videos because they were cringe.

'But when I saw other people who tube-feed share what they're going through, I was like, why don't I do it? I have the material to show the world. I can spread awareness. People really don't know about it. Even if one person learns something, that's a win for me. So I just started sharing stuff.'

The first video Deren posted was of him setting up a feed. It went viral. 'Everybody was commenting, like, what's that? Is that how he eats? Do you get hungry? Everyone was being so encouraging, so supportive,' he recalls.

But initially, Deren wasn't confident or comfortable with his tube. When he

/ feature

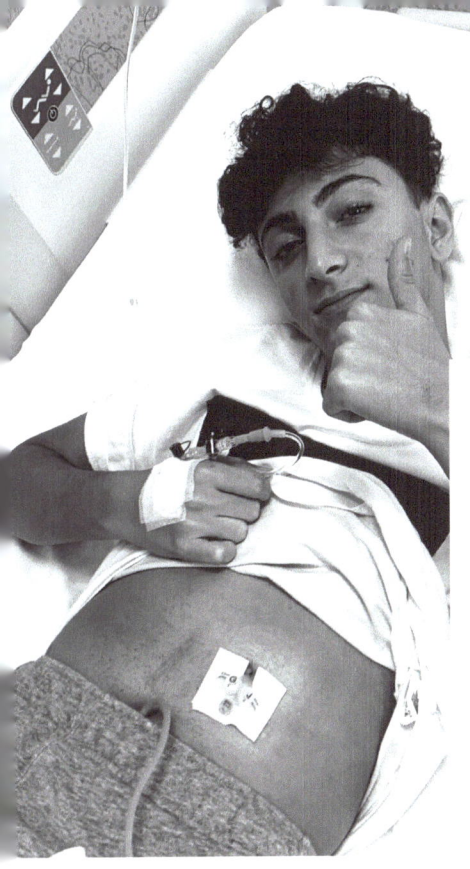

Deren Kıralp

Summer came and Deren started going to the beach. He'd transitioned to a surgical 'dangler' (long) tube, meaning he'd have to plaster it to his body. 'It looked really absurd because the plaster was white. My full abdomen was covered in white. People would look,' Deren says.

'One of my friends at the time said, "give me a tube and I will plaster my abdomen, so when people look at you, they can look at me too. There's no need to be shy or embarrassed". Of course got his NJ (nasojejunal) tube, he resolved that 'this is going to be who I am for a while', but ended up needing to continue tube-feeding. In those first few months, Deren didn't leave home and stopped going to school.

'I was really not ready for how to do the feeds outside,' he says. 'How would I manage?'

After a while, Deren came to the conclusion that he couldn't stay home anymore because, frankly, he 'was really bored'.

The first outing he had was to visit a friend, but as with many firsts, it had its challenges.

'I didn't have a real feed bag, those that have the hooks, so I just used a normal bag, but the pump was alarming at me,' says Deren. 'So next time, I just brought my pole. Then we started slowly going out with friends. Very slowly, though. I got used to people's looks.'

I didn't let her do that, but it was really sweet of her to say.'

Now Deren feels differently about his tube – comfortable even. His main piece of advice is to not be embarrassed, but to 'be confident'. However, he also concedes that advice 'doesn't really work'.

'As much as people tell you it's OK, people look. You still get shy,' he says. 'So I'm probably not going to say that as advice but I would say that with time those looks and stares will get better for you. They won't stop, but you won't feel them as much and you won't be embarrassed or be shy.'

The thought of tube-feeding is still daunting to me. The idea of not consuming food the 'usual' way will be something I will need to adapt to. But that's like anyone with any type of change. It takes time.

As I learnt from Jess and Deren, anyone can take something they've done forever one way – like eating – and find a new, just as fulfilling (and filling) way to achieve it. Also, the internet isn't all doom and gloom, it's also a place for community and shared learning.

Before we end our chat, Jess says: 'Even if you don't have a diagnosis or a tube yet, you can go and join those communities. They understand that it's a long, tedious and difficult process, and they'll back you the whole way. They may never meet you in real life, but they will be there for you. If there was ever any community to take that plunge with, it would be the tubie community.'

> "With time those looks, those stares will get better for you. They won't stop, but you won't feel them as much and you won't be embarrassed or be shy."

 Follow Kate's work @saidkatethomas

the blend. 39

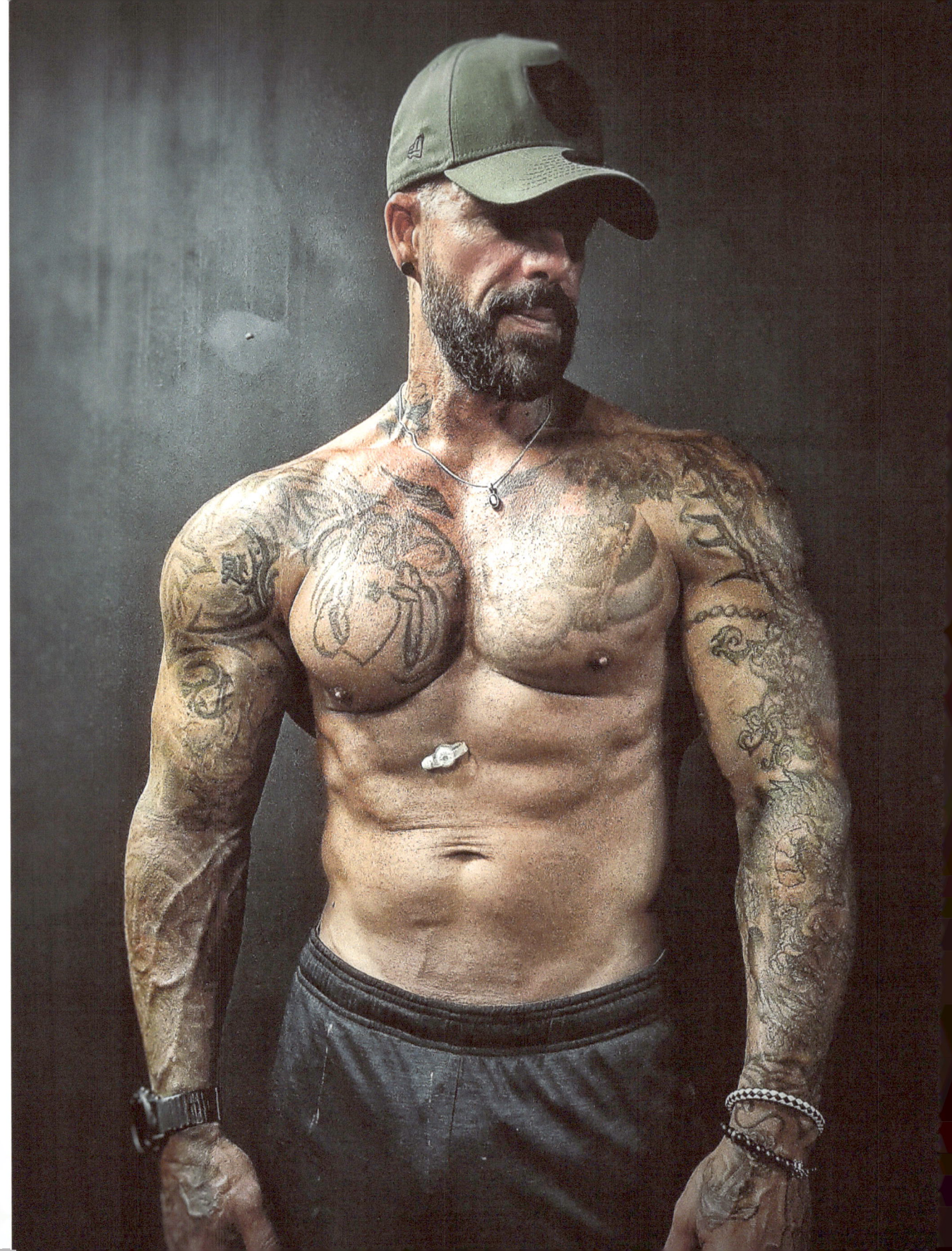

/ personal accounts

Strong stomach

Told he'd be eternally tethered to a feeding pump, Pedro Relvas spent the next two decades kicking that prognosis to the curb. Here, the South African-born, Brisbane-based body-sculpt athlete and coach shares how he's made tube-feeding work for him.

How did a gastrostomy (G) tube come into your life? When I was 25 years old I had surgery to remove a brain tumour. After that surgery I had paralysis of my glossopharyngeal nerve, which meant I couldn't swallow so the doctors had to put a tube in. I remember them telling me that I'd have to walk around with a feeding pump. I refused the pump and used syringes to feed from the start. I was on commercial formula for the first couple of years.

Did that formula sit well with you? Look, to be honest, that formula keeps you alive but I just wasn't able to get my weight back. I had so many negative side-effects, especially energy-wise. Most importantly it impacted my moods. I was not happy. So I got stubborn and decided, if I'm the one who's sick, I want to take care of myself and make my own choices, because I have to live with the consequences. Then came a long period of trial and error with blends.

How did you find your own way to this kind of diet? I've got a degree in neuropsychology and neuroscience tells us that we actually have three brains – in our head, heart and gut. If we look after our stomach, we can improve our mental wellness. Psychologists and psychotherapists are now treating patients through nutrition rather than pharmacology and I think we all need to be more focused on this. It sucks eating with a tube – of course it does. But it also sucks living with back pain or headaches. We all have our things that suck, we just don't want them to suck so much. And giving people who are tube-fed real, organic, unprocessed food makes a world of difference. It makes a world of difference for any person. >>

the blend.

My son is non-speaking so I'm always curious to know, when you are tube-fed, how long after you start a meal does it feel like you're filling up? It takes a while for my brain to register that my body's got food in it, so I've got a little bit of a cheat. If I'm at home I'll actually chew food while I'm tube-feeding and then spit it out into a bucket. I could be injecting a healthy meal and chewing on a pizza. So I get the best of both worlds.

You've got a great attitude toward tube-feeding, but at 25, when you discovered this was how you'd be eating, I'd imagine that was pretty crap. The hardest part about it was the visual aspect. I remember the first day that they put the PEG [percutaneous endoscopic gastrostomy] tube in, and my ex-wife – at the time she was my girlfriend – and my dad were with me. When they were asked to clean the tube, both of them had a really negative reaction. Which is normal. We're all human and not all of us can deal with a tube coming out of a stomach.

I remember getting really frustrated at that point and saying, 'all right, you guys leave' and I got the nurse to show me how to clean it. From then on I started to take control.

It was also hard to navigate the social aspect. The toughest thing for me – and it still happens to this day – is I don't really get invited out for dinner. People don't want to make me uncomfortable, so they just kind of back off.

So I tried to have some fun with my tube-feeding. I came up with a few party tricks. My friends would syringe different flavoured proteins into me and I'd guess what they were.

So you can actually taste the food when it goes in? It has a little bit of an aftertaste – at least in my experience. The best way to describe it is, you know when you've had a really big meal and then about 20 minutes later, you can kind of still taste it? That's what it feels like.

My friends became more and more supportive but I still deal with people's

> "My friends became more and more supportive but I still deal with people's assumptions. When some people see me feeding in the gym, their first thought is, 'oh, he's taking steroids'."

assumptions. When some people see me feeding in the gym, their first thought is, 'oh, he's taking steroids', because they see a massive syringe. But when people actually ask, 'what's that?' I have the chance to explain and they understand. Some people even say, 'you're so lucky, that's why you look the way you look'.

And the truth is, I probably wouldn't be as disciplined today had I not had my tube. I also wouldn't know as much today had I not had it. It's part of who I am – but it's not everything.

It certainly isn't. You've got two kids, haven't you? Yes, my son is 18 and my daughter is 14. They're into health and fitness as well. Most kids want to be in the gym because they want to look good, but with my son and my daughter, I really enforce that if you feel good, you will always look good. So we focus on feeling good.

Nowadays, many of my personal training clients choose to feed the same way I do. A lot of them will blend their meals and drink them throughout the day. They find that the blended food doesn't sit in their stomach as long and they process it easier, so they love it.

Like you say – nutrition has so much to do with feeling good. When we switched from formula to blended food, my kid got his sparkle back. I can only imagine what it's like when your child needs to tube-feed. I often feel lucky because I'm going through it, so I can figure it out for myself. In your situation and with your son not being able to speak, you must wonder, what is he feeling? Am I hurting him? Is he still hungry? It must be really hard. >>

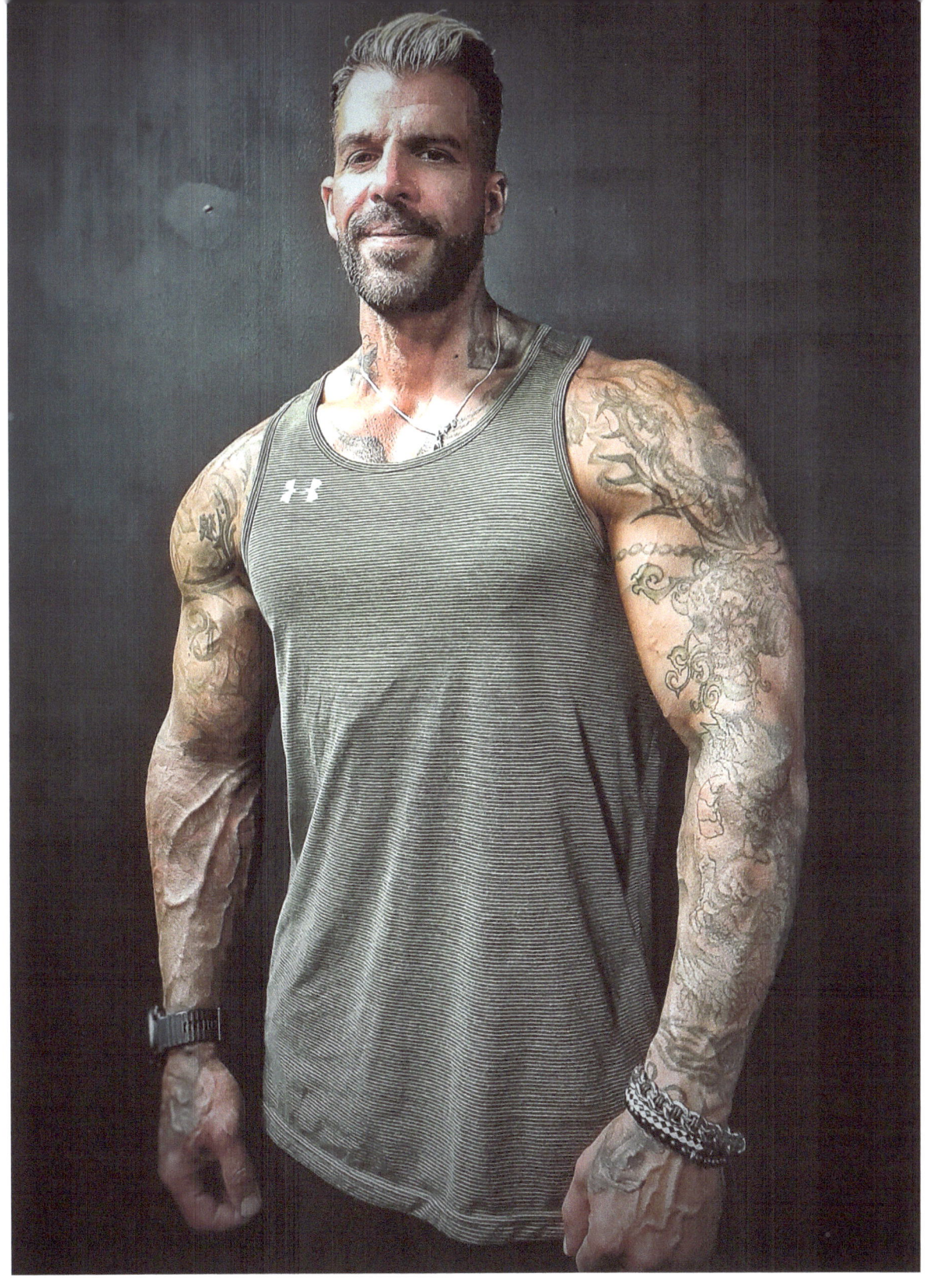

But with your understanding of your son and your awareness of his nonverbal cues – and I'm a big believer in energetic communication, as well – you must be so in tune. There will be things that you see, sense, and just know.

You really get it, Pedro, and those are some beautiful words for parents. What about adults who are new to tube-feeding and feeling like it's the end of their work life, social life, sex life... The end of your sex life – that's something I was worried about. After my divorce I thought, how do I meet someone new? I opened myself up and even started online dating for a bit and met a couple of people there who were put off by the idea of my tube.

I found myself feeling quite rejected by it. And then I thought, you know what? I don't think I would even relate to you as a friend if that's your perception of someone, so why am I taking this so personally? That little bit of negativity woke me up to the fact that I hadn't fully accepted myself and I was able to release that.

For the record, you have a supportive partner now, don't you? Yes I do, she's amazing. She's a down to earth, easy-going person. And even when I wake up at night and have to spit, it doesn't phase her. In fact, she often compliments me and says that her own awareness of her health and fitness is because she lives with me. I was really, really lucky to find her, but I often tease and say she was very lucky to find me.

It goes both ways! What advice do you have for anyone who is new to tube-feeding? When I talk to people who are tube-fed I always remind them, you don't work for the tube. Make it work for you. I'm stuck in this situation, so how can I make the best of it? Take advice, of course, but make sure you take control and make the choices.

The parents who are dealing with this, who are open and actively searching for answers, are inspirational to me because that's what makes the change. Your son is going to be an amazing person because of your attitude to this process. And at the same time, it's because of your son that you've been opened up to so many different possibilities.

To anyone who's new to tube-feeding I say it's going to be tough, but at the end of the day, it's going to be yours.

> "Take advice, of course, but make sure you take control and make the choices."

@wolfpepe
@FitnMeaningful

Professional perspectives.

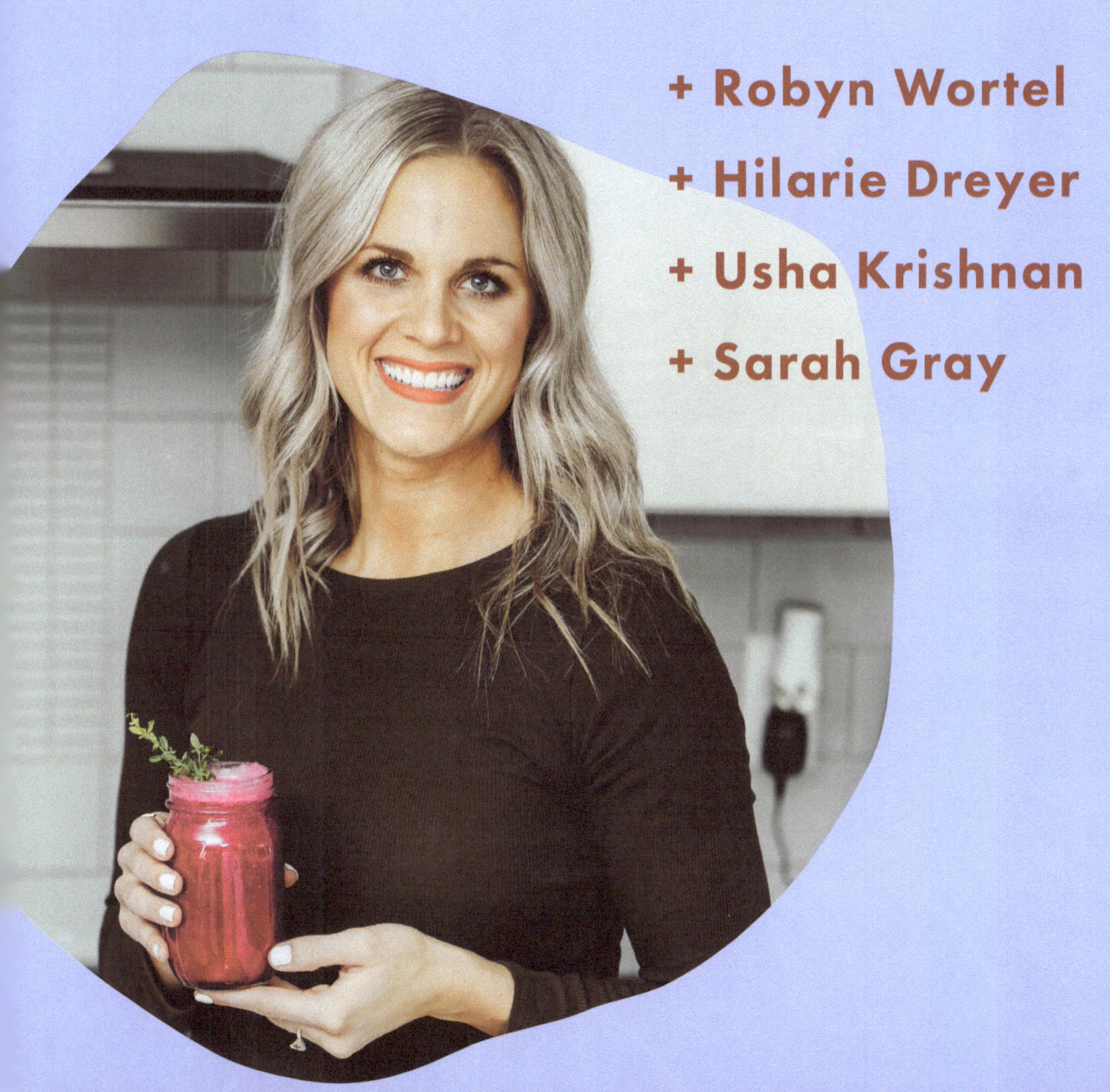

+ Robyn Wortel
+ Hilarie Dreyer
+ Usha Krishnan
+ Sarah Gray

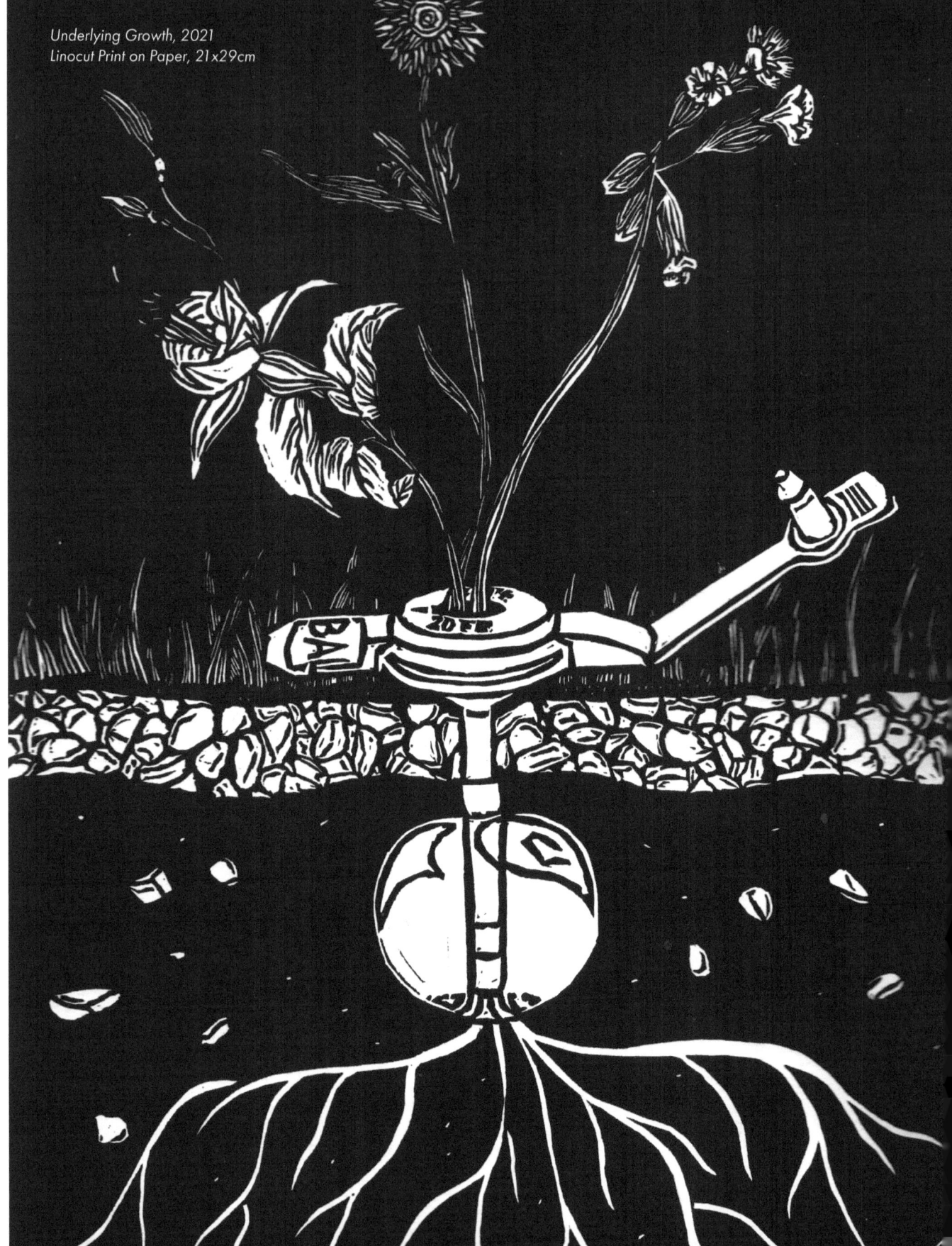
Underlying Growth, 2021
Linocut Print on Paper, 21x29cm

/ feature

G-tube feeding 101

New to the great, life-changing device that is a gastrostomy tube? Take note of these top tips.

Artwork: Kathryn Lean

Robyn Wortel was a registered nurse and is now the clinical education specialist at Avanos, maker of the MIC-KEY G-tube and many other nifty enteral-feeding devices. For more than 20 years, Robyn's job has been to educate doctors, nurses and caregivers who are introducing people to tube-feeding.

'They are the first line of contact for parents and family members and you would hope that the information you share with them gets shared with the people who need it,' says Robyn. 'But then, there's so much else going on in those lives, so how much can you take in?'

In truth, there's a flood of finicky details to contend with when a tube enters your world. So it's handy to have some pointers in print, straight from an expert.

'Oh no, no,' Robyn protests when described – accurately – in this fashion. 'You know what they say about an expert? That an ex is a has-been and a spurt is a drip under pressure. If I've got some knowledge to share, I'm always happy to share it.' >>

the blend.   47

And with that, Robyn offers her best tips for getting a grip on G-tubes:

DON'T FEAR THE TUBE

It's OK. You can touch it. You can feel it. It shouldn't be painful for your loved one at all and if it is, there might be something wrong. Maybe the fit isn't right. You should be able to turn or rotate the tube and the skin disc should sit just a little bit above the skin. Think of this like putting on a pair of jeans before you've had lunch. You need a little bit of space there because there's a little bit of expansion as a tummy fills.

PREPARE FOR CHANGE

A G-tube goes in looking white but it never stays white. The colour it changes to is very much dependent on what food and medication is being fed through the tube. Those things colour a tube and they also colour the water that you use to fill the balloon. This is especially noticeable if you're doing blenderised feeds and using highly colourful foods like beetroot, spinach or carrots.

TEST THE WATER

The silicone in the balloon is a semi-permeable membrane, which is why you get variation in colour in the water and also why you get a little bit of volume loss. You can put 5ml in today and next week check it and it's 4ml. We recommend checking the water every week, but you might only need to check every two or three weeks if you've got consistent care and can gauge what's happening. It's really important to trust your gut here.

GET THE FIT RIGHT

If you don't have the tube fitted correctly, you're going to have problems. Especially with the low-profile MIC-KEY but also if you've got a long tube, the disc that sits on the skin needs to sit at 2-3mm above skin level. If it's sitting higher, you're going to have friction and changes in the position of the tube. It's going to affect the shape of the stoma and it's going to allow gastric leakage to escape.

Friction creates hypergranulation – a ballooning of highly fragile, very moist 'proud flesh' that bleeds easily and can be painful. If you don't have friction, you probably won't get that type of granulation.

> "Do whatever you can do to make tube-feeding as normal as possible. The most basic need of any parent or carer is being able to feed the one you love."

KEEP THE STOMA SITE DRY

I love the button pads that Stacey at Tubie Fun makes. But whatever you might put around your stoma, if it gets wet, you need to change it. Because even though it's got a wicking material in it, if it's moist and it sits on the skin, you're going to end up with soggy skin which is more likely to break down and create problems. Some stomas will always have some moisture and others are perfectly dry. It's very much person dependent.

NORMALISE, NORMALISE, NORMALISE

Do whatever you can do to make tube-feeding as normal as possible. The most basic need of any parent or carer is being able to feed the one you love. If you can do that in whatever way it takes, however it works, and you can see that your loved one is thriving, then you're doing the best job you can. So have a pat on the back for that.

/ feature

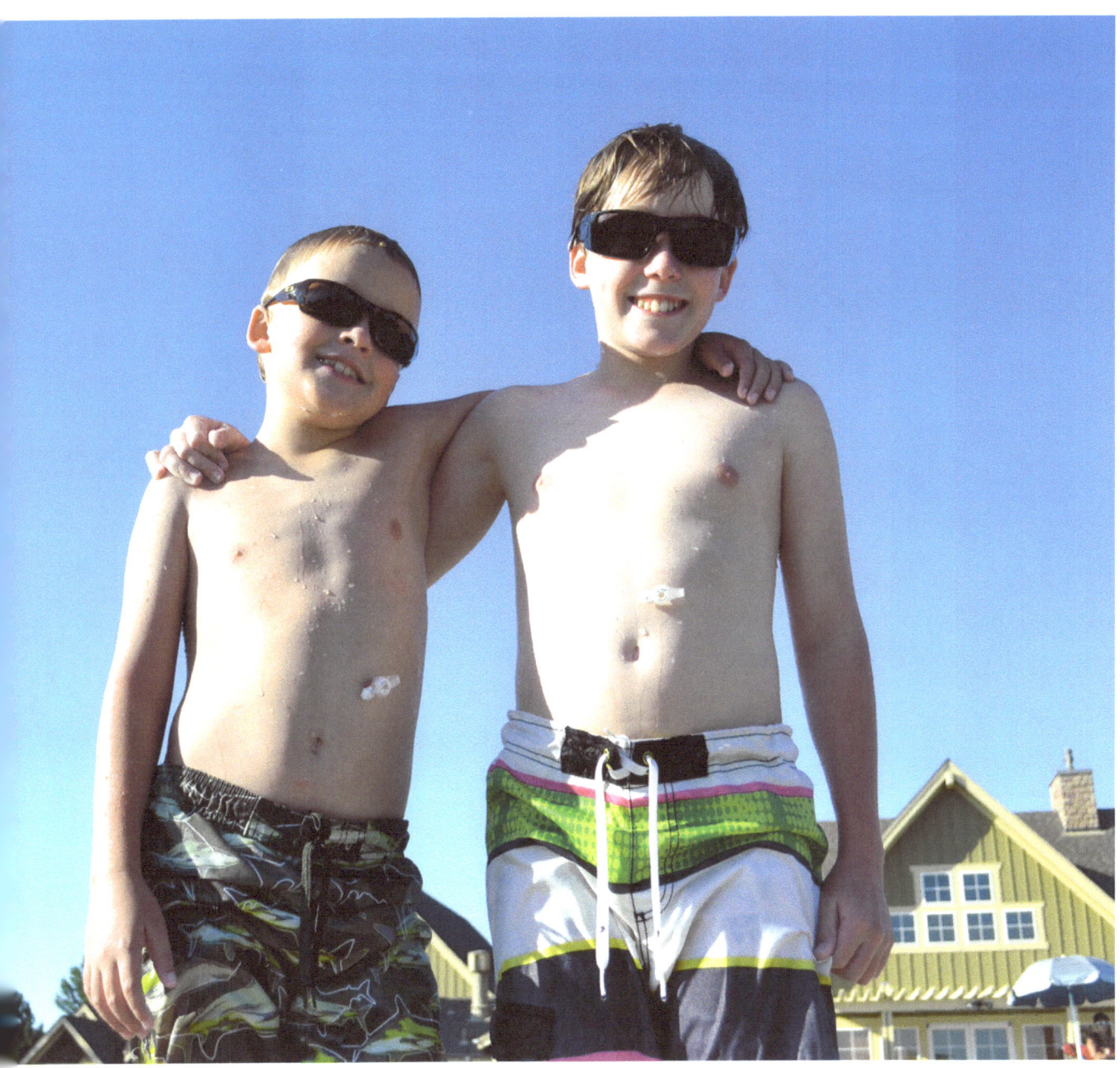

AVANOS

This article was made in partnership with Avanos. For easily digestible information about tube-feeding at any age and any stage, visit TubeFed by Avanos at tubefed.com.au.

the blend.

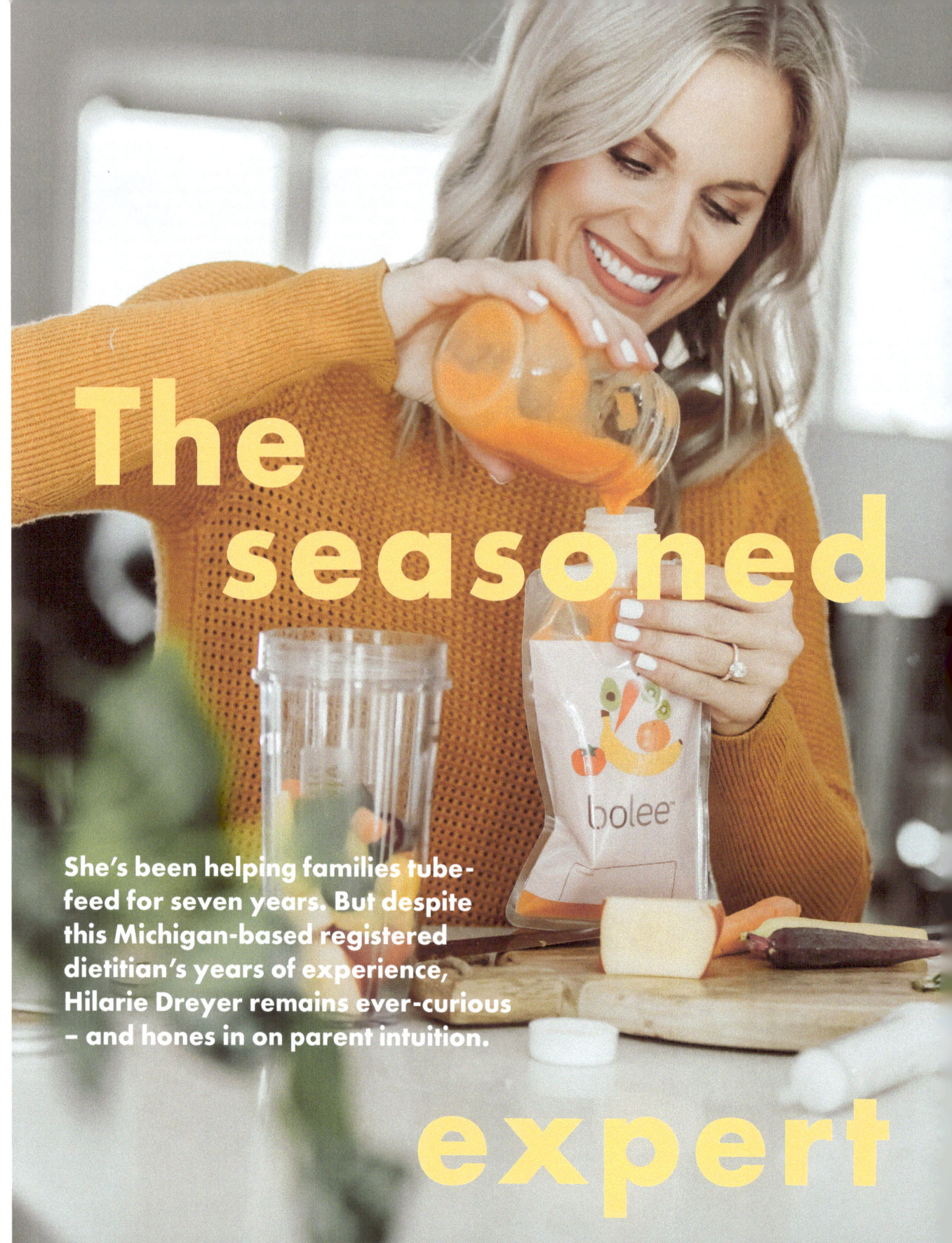

The seasoned expert

She's been helping families tube-feed for seven years. But despite this Michigan-based registered dietitian's years of experience, Hilarie Dreyer remains ever-curious – and hones in on parent intuition.

/ professional perspectives

What's your first memory of food? Corn days. I grew up on a farm and my dad had a big garden with lots of ears of corn. We would spend two days as a family husking it, cooking it, bagging it and freezing it for the winter. As a kid I remember thinking, 'oh my gosh, this is the worst thing ever'. But I grew to appreciate it. Nowadays my fiancé and I have a big garden and enjoy canning and preserving our own food.

When did you realise that food – and the science behind it – was something you wanted to pursue professionally? I kind of fell into this career. I actually started out as a nurse and then I went to a fashion school, which wasn't for me at all. I really like to work with people and I also really like the science behind metabolism and how the human body digests nutrition. Someone suggested I become a dietitian and that's what I did.

At what point did tube-feeding become an interest? I was always interested in paediatrics and critical care, but when I found out how little interaction you have with people in that setting, I became more interested in helping families in outpatient clinics. When I moved home after my internship there weren't any openings at the children's hospital, so I started home visiting with a lot of kids who were tube-fed, which spurred my appreciation for the parent perspective.

Being in homes and seeing how often families were given recommendations that didn't work for them or align with their goals, that was a game-changer for me. After doing this for two years I moved into a hospital setting and worked with thousands of tube-feeding kids. Then in 2021, I started my private service to better support families with blended diets.

When you say you went into people's homes and saw that tube-feeding wasn't working, what do you mean? Well, I'm a big advocate for 'fed is best' and 'all formula fits', and using a commercial formula is best for some people. But I would see these kids get sent home on a regimen that wasn't well tolerated or didn't make sense for the family. I learnt that we need to be more realistic with families about what is actually working for them.

What got me more into real food is the digestive issues that people are having on the commercial formulas. These kids would be going through so many medications and so many procedures for their digestive issues and we'd never address what we're feeding them. I'd see them after three years of them going through every specialist and they'd still be on the same formula. Why haven't we tried a real food-based product?

> "Being in homes and seeing how often families were given recommendations that didn't work for them or align with their goals, that was a game-changer for me."

There's still some resistance to blended feeds in the Australian medical sector. How widely accepted is this diet in the US? The last clinic I was working in was pro-blends, but I wouldn't say this diet is widely accepted. It's not that dietitians and health providers think it's a bad way to feed, they just don't have the knowledge and time to figure it out. That's where I was, too, and that's what led me to teach myself home blending and start a private practice. Families need way more support than we give them in the clinical setting, which often provides minimal guidance on blending nuances. >>

the blend.

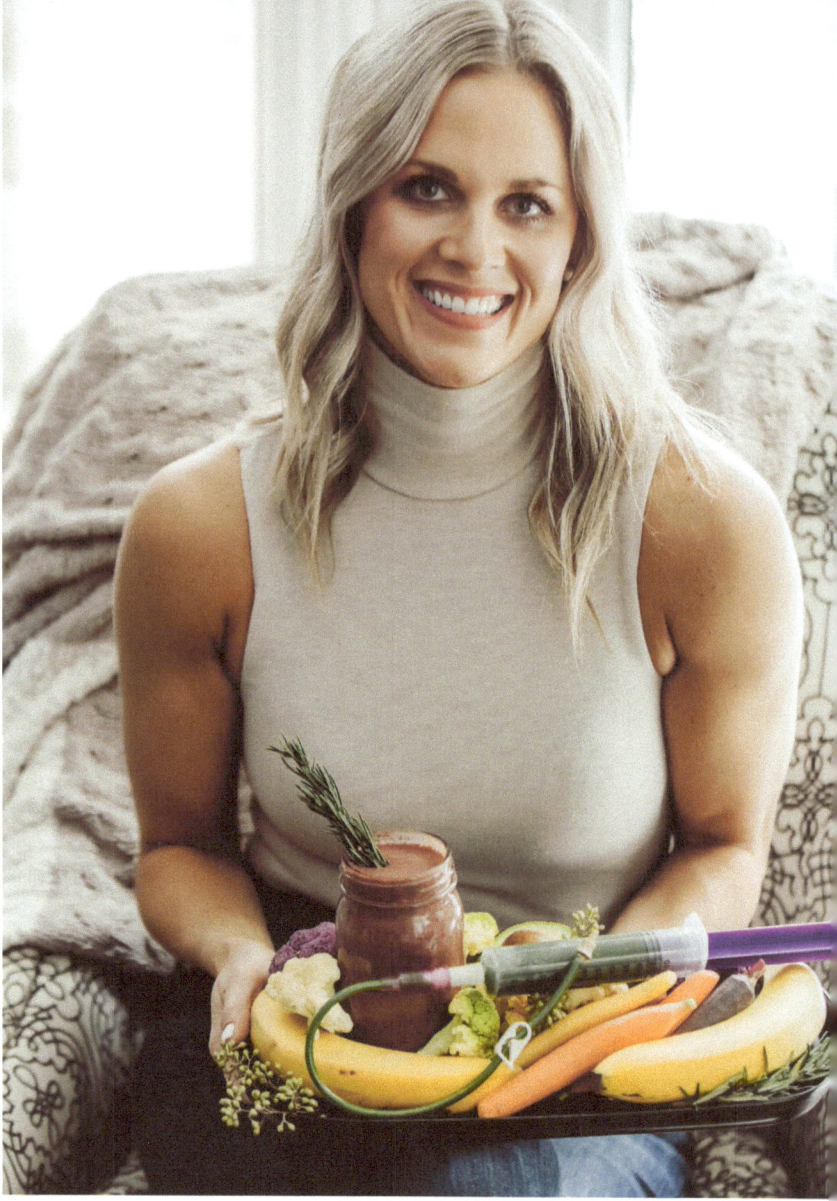

In a lot of places I've worked we were prioritising numbers over patient care. When you're pushed to see so many patients it's a lot easier to prescribe a commercial formula regimen than it is to teach people about blends. It's a bad cycle and families are accepting a suboptimal state of health for their child because it's all they've ever known.

Your work philosophy is, 'instead of me telling you what to do, you can tell me what you want to do and I will support you in that'. Where does this approach stem from? I feel like I can learn just as much from parents as they can learn from me. If not more, honestly. It can be intimidating to put myself out there and say 'teach me what you know', because I'm supposed to be the expert, right? But in order to bridge some of these gaps between medical professionals and parents, we really need to work together and learn from each other.

I'm imagining you encounter a lot of emotions from families who are new to this space. How do you support parents who are struggling to come to terms with their child needing to tube-feed? I think that a lot of the problem is that, often, parents feel unheard. So I try to be a listening ear, take in their perspectives and hold space for how they're feeling. I also think it's important for families to realise they aren't alone in this. That's why I've set up my virtual program, where families are able to connect in weekly group Zoom calls. Through this we build community and learn from each other.

I also love sharing podcasts that help families feel supported, and my favourite one is The Rare Life. That podcast provides solidarity for these families in ways I can't because I don't know what it's like to go through what they're going through.

Even with professional guidance from someone like you, getting tube-feeding right is still about trial and error – and trying not to freak out – right? I always say to parents, this is what I think is going to happen, but if it doesn't, it's OK. We'll figure it out together and it's going to be fine. And as we go, you'll start to gain confidence because I'm giving you permission to try things, see what works and what doesn't, and you have my support and guidance along the way.

Hilarie's six tips for top-notch blends

1. For nutritional variety, be sure to mix up what foods you're blending. Rotating through different coloured fruits and vegetables will provide a wide variety of vitamins and minerals. Switch up your protein, grain and healthy fat sources. If your blended meals are limited in variety or you need to avoid whole food groups, you're likely missing out on important nutrients and supplementation may be needed. Be sure to discuss this with your healthcare team.
2. Storage containers should be airtight and nonporous to prevent the blended food from spoiling. Deli containers and mason jars are great options for storing blends as they are freezer, microwave and dishwasher safe. I also love deli containers because they stack well in the freezer for optimal storage.
3. Aim for a thin, pancake-batter consistency with your blended meals. This may seem thick if you're used to formula, but it's the higher viscosity (thickness) of blended meals that has been clinically shown to help with digestive issues like reflux and vomiting.
4. Warming food slightly before feeding can really help with digestion and tolerance. Use a warm-water bath rather than the microwave to avoid uneven heating.
5. Use syringes with an O-ring silicone plunger rather than a rubber plunger. The O-ring silicone plunger doesn't wear out or expand with use, making it much easier on your hands to push the food through. My favourite is the Basik O-ring syringe, most families say these last at least four months.
6. Don't be afraid to add herbs and spices to your blended food. There are so many health benefits to herbs and spices and they are an easy thing to add to a blend. Try some turmeric for anti-inflammatory benefits, ginger for gastrointestinal issues, or oregano which is high in antioxidants.

Find Hilarie's strawberry shortcake overnight oats blend recipe on page 116.

---

 blendedtubefeeding.com

 @blendedtubefeeding

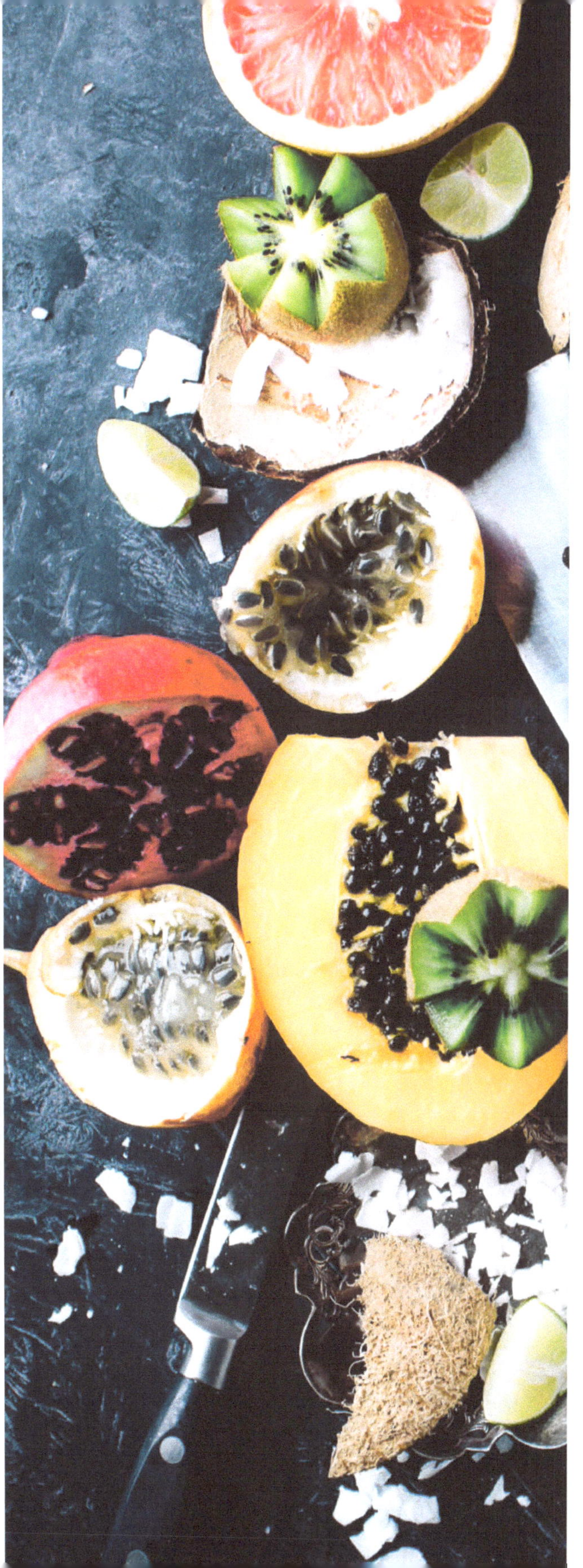

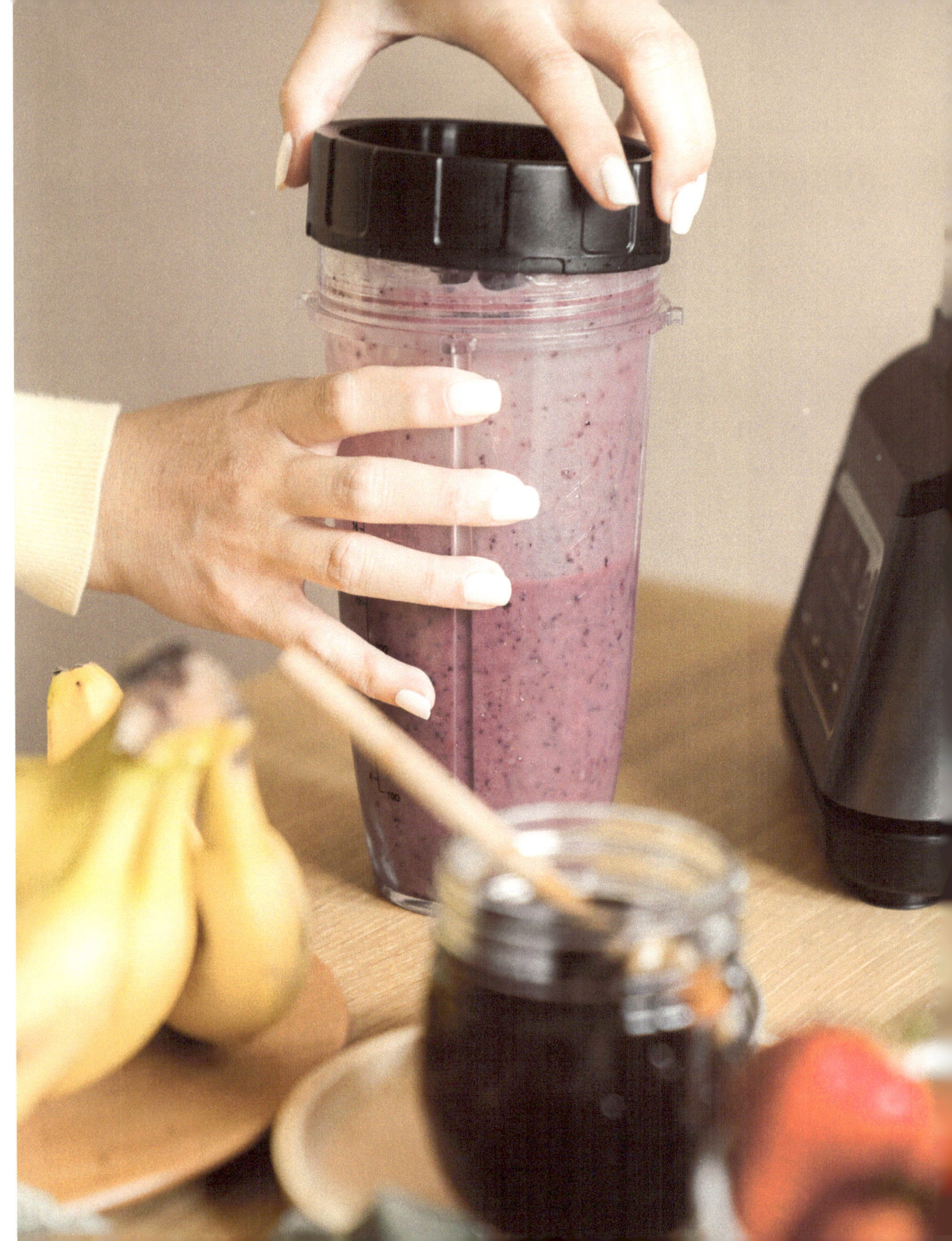

/ professional perspectives

The gut healer

Paediatric gastroenterologist Usha Krishnan is passionate about tummies. She was one of the experts who developed the AuSPEN consensus statement for blenderised tube-feeds, so who better to ask how this diet is changing the enteral-feeding space.

Why are stomachs your chosen specialty? As a paediatric gastroenterologist, the stomach is an integral part of my area of specialisation. But I've always been passionate about food, nutrition and children's growth because it impacts not only on the gastrointestinal system, but overall wellbeing and quality of life – and not only of the child, but of their whole family.

What are your earliest memories of food and family? I was born in India and Indian food is very diverse, colourful and tasty. My earliest memories are of my mum cooking different kinds of foods in the kitchen and me hanging on to her, following her around and trying to see what she was doing.

Why did blended feeds become an area of interest for you? A significant proportion of the children that I look after have enteral feeding and although commercial formulas are nutritionally complete and help a child grow, I was increasingly hearing children – or their parents – saying they were having side-effects from the standard formulas.

Yes, they were putting on weight, but they might be complaining of tummy pain. They could have bloating, diarrhoea or constipation. They might be vomiting, gagging and retching. Do we really need children to be on something that is making them unwell in other ways, even though they might be putting on weight?

This is one area where innovation has been led by parents more than doctors. I started hearing about real blended food from parents and that stimulated me to read and learn more about it so I could help my patients. In the last two to three years, half of the parents I see are asking me about blended feeds.

Arlo, my son, was orally eating real food right up until his G-tube was put in – but we got sent home from hospital with a carton of commercial formula. Why is this happening? It really shouldn't be happening. One of the dietitians in our hospital did a study that found parents saying 'we got more information from the internet than we did from our doctors and dietitians'. I know we should be helping you and supporting you. >>

And hopefully under the new consensus guidelines for the use of blenderised tube feeds which have come out from Australasian Society of Parenteral and Enteral Nutrition (AuSPEN), parents will feel empowered to tell the doctors and dietitians, 'we want to do this'.

We are educating the dietitians, too. And as they are learning more about it, they're feeling more comfortable prescribing it. This is why we need more research into it – and that's what we're trying to do at AuSPEN. We're trying to get more funding to do more research, because if doctors and dietitians understand more about why blends work, they'll be more willing to support this diet.

What evidence does exist around the benefits of blended feeds?

We recently did a study where we compared a group of kids on blends to a group of kids on commercial formula and we found that both were equally nutritionally complete. But for the kids on blends, their gastrointestinal problems and quality of life was better, the microbiome [community of microorganisms living in the gut] was richer and more diverse and they had less inflammation in their bowels.

However, I should mention that we did find that they'd need more calories to maintain the same rate of growth, so blends weren't for everyone. But we also discovered that you don't necessarily need to be exclusively in one group or the other. Even a diet of 25 per cent blends was enough to reduce symptoms and still help maintain growth.

Is there progress being made in the commercial formula space for kids who are limited to this diet?

Absolutely. Everything's about the microbiome and if you have a richer, more diverse microbiome, it's better for your overall health. So they're trying to add prebiotics and probiotics and reduce preservatives in the commercial formula space, too.

The team at AuSPEN published the blenderised tube-feeds consensus statement, what's next?

We're also trying to develop a web-based app for blenderised tube-feeds. The idea is that you tell the app what you've put in your blender and it tells you the exact nutritional information for your meal. I hope we're able to get funding to develop this app – it could be a fantastic resource.

What advice do you have for families who are keen to try blends?

You need close supervision with a knowledgeable dietitian to be sure that your child is meeting nutritional requirements. Some studies have shown you need 120 to 150 per cent extra calories on a blended diet to maintain the same rate of weight gain that you would on a standard formula. So parents need to be willing to work creatively with their medical team and dietitian.

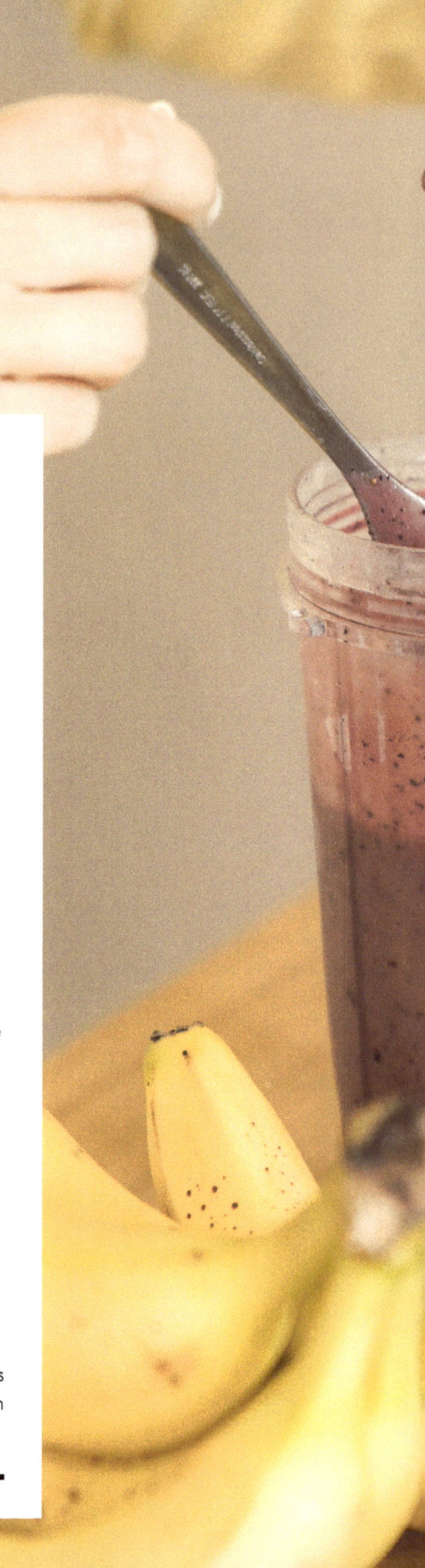

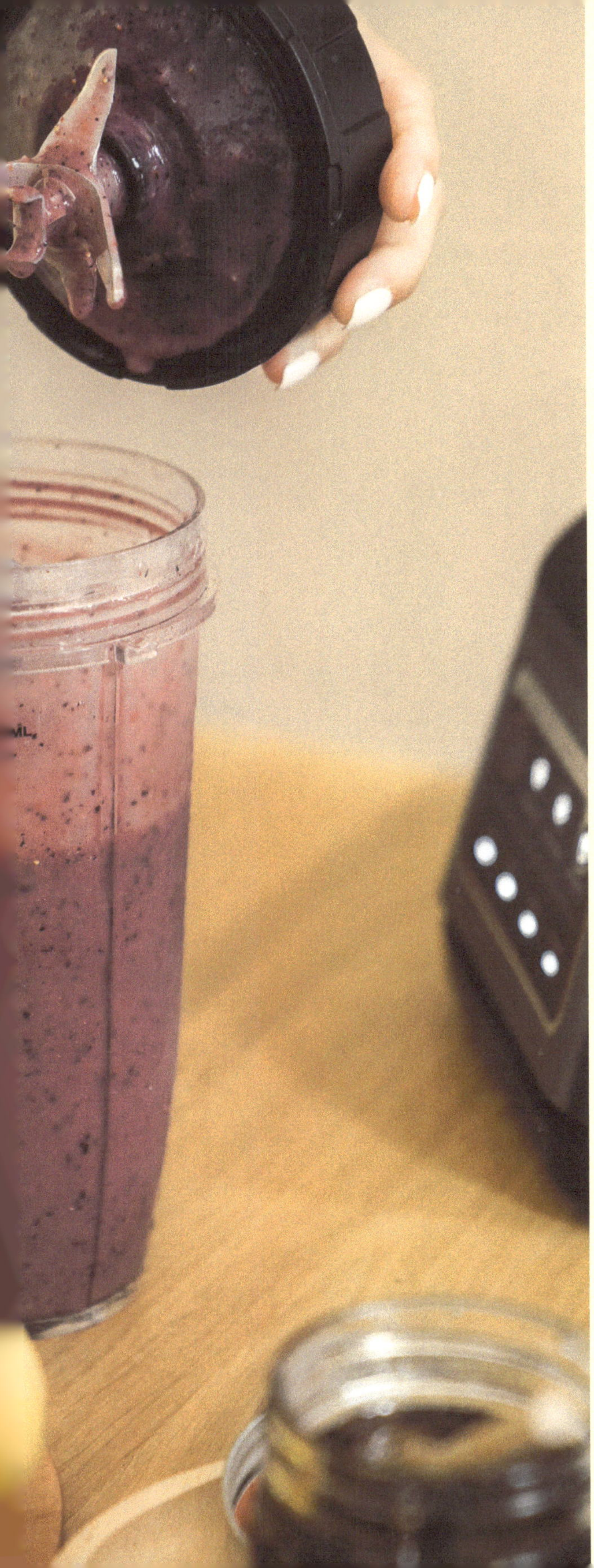

/ professional perspectives

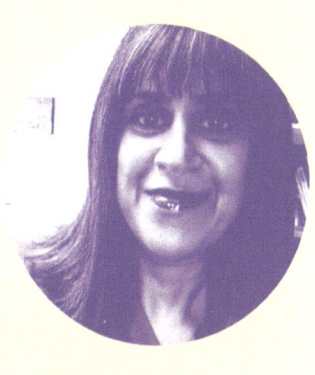

Usha's pros and cons of a blenderised diet

PROS

+ It might help with abdominal pain, nausea, vomiting, gagging, retching, bloating, wind, constipation and diarrhoea.
+ Children on this diet reportedly seem happier in themselves and feel more part of the family during meal times.
+ It might mean less infections, hospitalisations and admissions.

CONS

- It's not recommended for children on continuous feeds, those on jejunal feeds, or those under six months of age.
- It might not suit people with very complex metabolic problems, multiple food allergies, or those who are immunosuppressed, because it's not prepared in a sterile environment.
- Very small tubes can get blocked. To avoid blockages you need to have a really good blender, which might be out of reach financially for some families.

the blend.

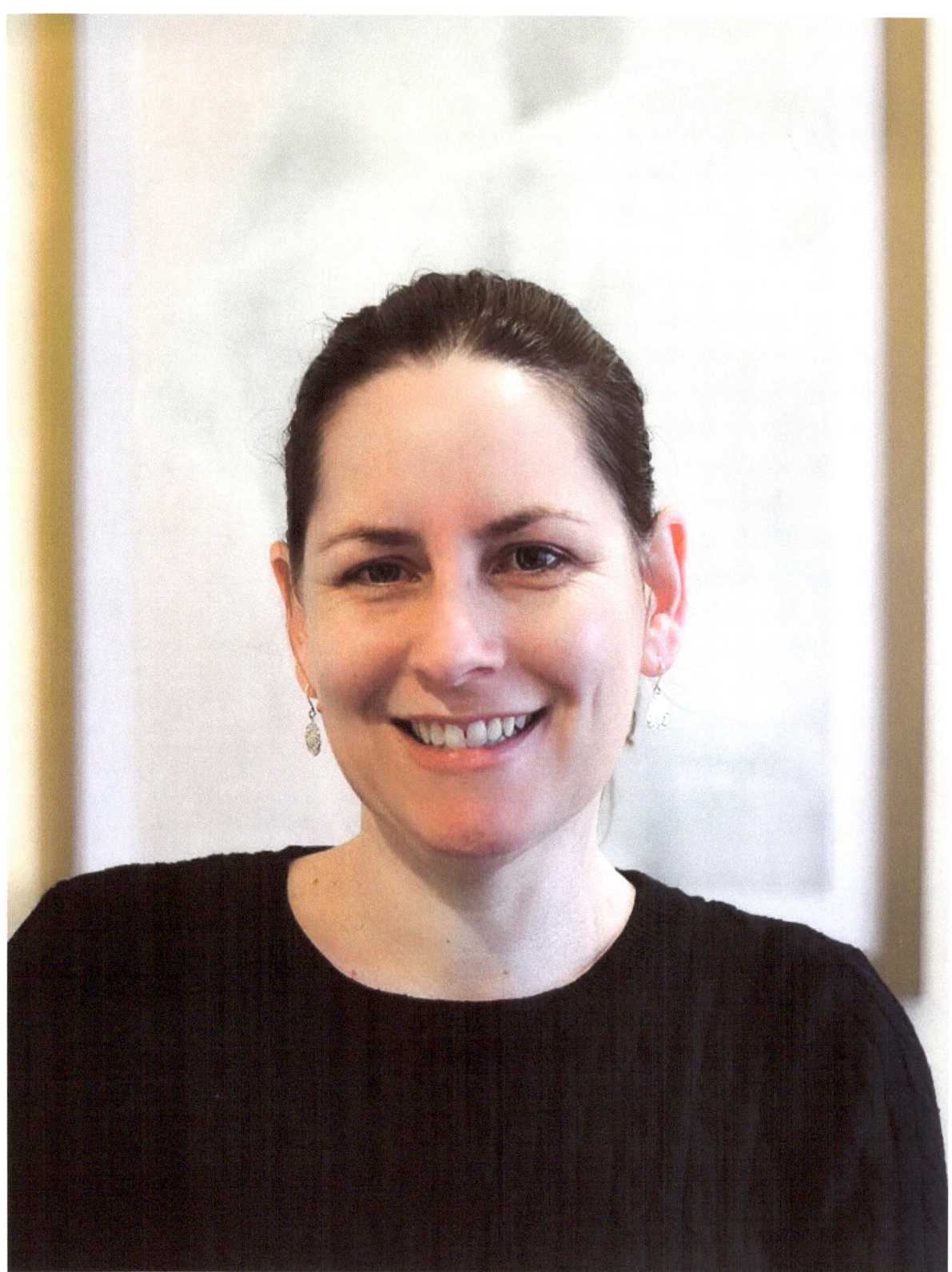

/ **professional perspectives**

The ultimate connector

When Sarah Gray's toddler was diagnosed with a chronic inflammatory condition and later began tube-feeding, the Sunshine Coast-based mother felt entirely alone. But rather than wallow and whinge, she rescued herself – and created a community for countless families like hers.

From four months of age, when my daughter, Bella, was failing to thrive, doctors started talking about the possibility of a feeding tube. At 18 months old we discovered she had eosinophilic oesophagitis (EoE) but she was still able to drink elemental formula, which meant we endured a very long decision-making process.

It's really hard to make the decision to get a tube when a child is capable of drinking. Bella would say, 'no, I'll drink more Mummy. Don't do it'.

It wasn't until age seven that Bella, herself, contributed to that decision. I remember watching a *60 Minutes* story about a girl who was dying from cancer. Bella came into the room and saw it and she said, 'Mummy, I look like her. Am I dying?'. As a mother, it's a heartbreaking thing to hear your child say. I think at that moment she realised how sick she was and she said she wanted to get the feeding tube that we had long talked about. It was such a relief, like a huge weight had finally been lifted. >>

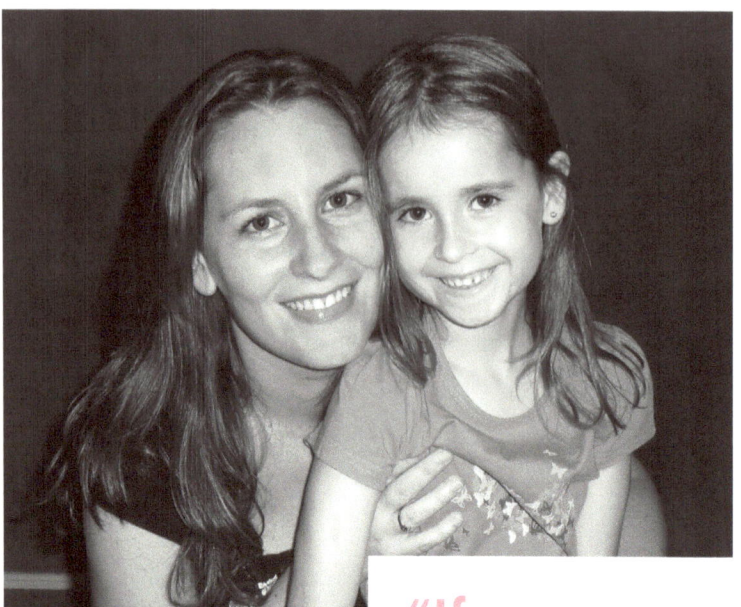
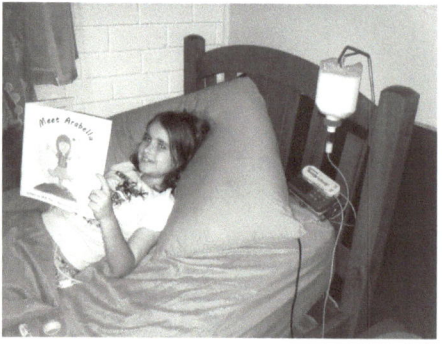

We let her dietitian and medical team know and everyone agreed it was the best thing to do. I only wish we'd come to that decision sooner. We had really struggled for many years because Bella was always a question mark. Will she tube-feed? No, she's doing OK. We'll keep plodding along. I remember I'd have to push her around in the pram with her sister, Olivia, who's two years younger. People thought they were twins, because they looked the same size.

Bella put on 8kg in the first year of having her feeding tube. She finally had energy. You don't realise you don't have energy until you have it. It was just remarkable the difference in her. And that made me regret even more not doing it sooner. That's part of the reason why I started raising awareness, because jeez, we need to remove that stigma around tube-feeding – the misconception that it's scary and something that's not done at home.

By the time Bella got her gastrostomy tube, I had already founded ausEE Inc.,

> "If you are new to tube-feeding, don't feel like you have to go through that alone. Find and connect with groups where you can share how you're feeling."

a charity raising awareness for eosinophilic diseases and was volunteering, together with Mercedez Hinchcliff, whose son Henry has EoE and was also on an elemental formula. This meant I already knew a lot of people and families who had children on elemental formula and a few who were tube-feeding, which was fortunate because once Bella got that tube put in, we were pretty much on our own.

The hospital gave us 500ml bottles for Bella's feeds and when the pump alarm would go off in the middle of the night, my husband and I would take turns getting up to make the next feed and switch it over. A year or two of this down the track, someone asked us, why don't you use the litre bottles? We were like, they have litre bottles? It's the little

things like that that no one really tells you at the start.

When a fellow mum of a child who was tube-fed, Kate Anderson, started the Facebook group AU tubie support, I joined. Every February, during Feeding Tube Awareness Week (FTAW) we would share a bunch of American resources until eventually it dawned on us – hang on, we're a whole country here, why can't we be doing this?

I contacted the Feeding Tube Awareness Foundation in America and asked if they would mind us launching a local FTAW campaign. They told us to go for it and so, from 2015 onwards, we've celebrated this week by informing and connecting Australia's tube-feeding community.

/ **professional perspectives**

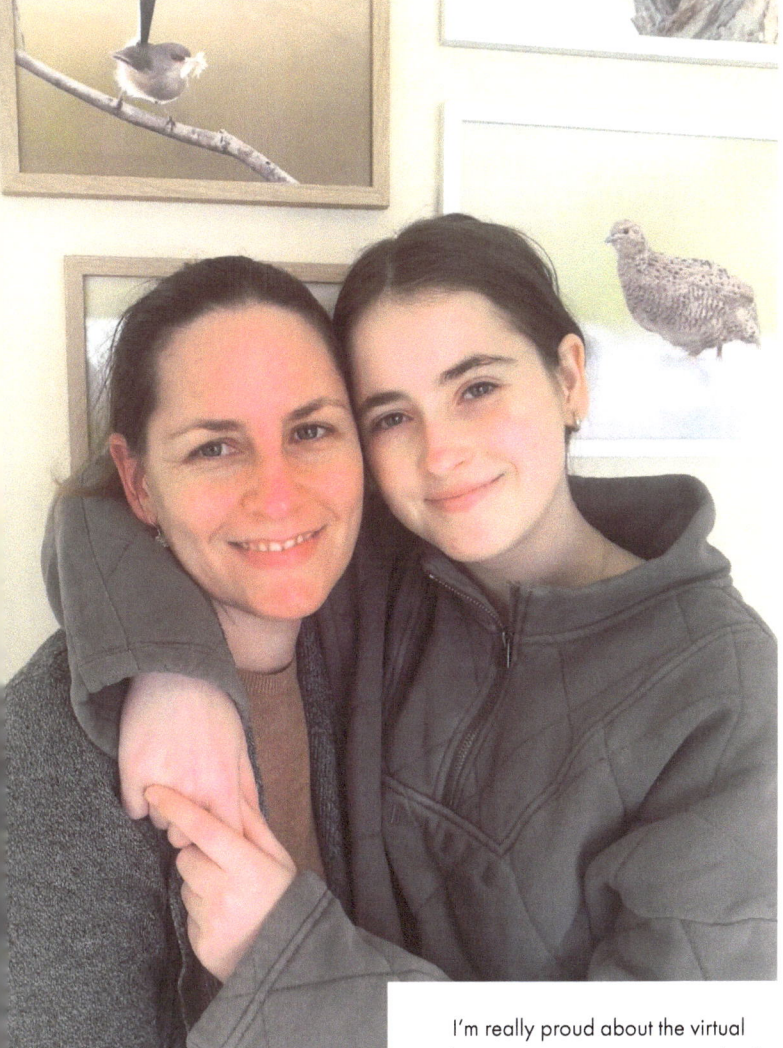

I'm really proud about the virtual education program we put together for FTAW last year. This year, landmarks across Australia and New Zealand will be lit up in purple and blue to mark the occasion. We keep notching things up a little higher every year, with the goal of bringing more people together.

Bella built our feeding tube awareness website, which is full of resources and links to services and social networks. We also run virtual support groups which connect around 3000 people in the EoE and tube-feeding community.

Bella no longer has her tube, but we like to think, once a tubie, always a tubie. Her EoE has been well managed for several years too, but that doesn't stop us from wanting to help people.

If you are new to tube-feeding, don't feel like you have to go through that alone. Find and connect with groups where you can share how you're feeling. Talk to your family about it, too. Try not to hide like I did at first, when I was crying myself to sleep every night.

I saw a psychologist at the time, only once, as I didn't connect with her because she didn't want me to talk about what Bella was going through. She wanted me to talk about me and kept saying, but what about self-care? I get that, but at the time, I needed someone to talk to about what I was going through with Bella.

She was a bit abrupt with me when she said: 'Well, surely you're not the only one going through this. You've just got to find those other people and then talk to them about it.'

That was an epiphany moment for me. It felt like the *Field of Dreams* movie with Kevin Costner – if you build it, they will come! So I took long-service leave from my job, started the ausEE Inc. charity and other families did – as Kevin Costner promised – come.

I remember a supervisor I once worked with saying, 'don't bring me a problem unless you're also bringing me a solution'. Well, this charity was my solution. Why was I complaining about there being no information out there for families like mine? Let's make that solution! And 13 years later, here we are.

 Visit ausee.org and feedingtubeaware.com.au for support, information and connection.

the blend.

YOUR COMPREHENSIVE TO ENTERAL FEEDING

BROUGHT TO YOU BY THE MAKERS OF MIC-KEY*

- Every Stage - Every Age
- Short Term to Long Term Feeding

tubefed.com.au
BY AVANOS

ONLINE GUIDE

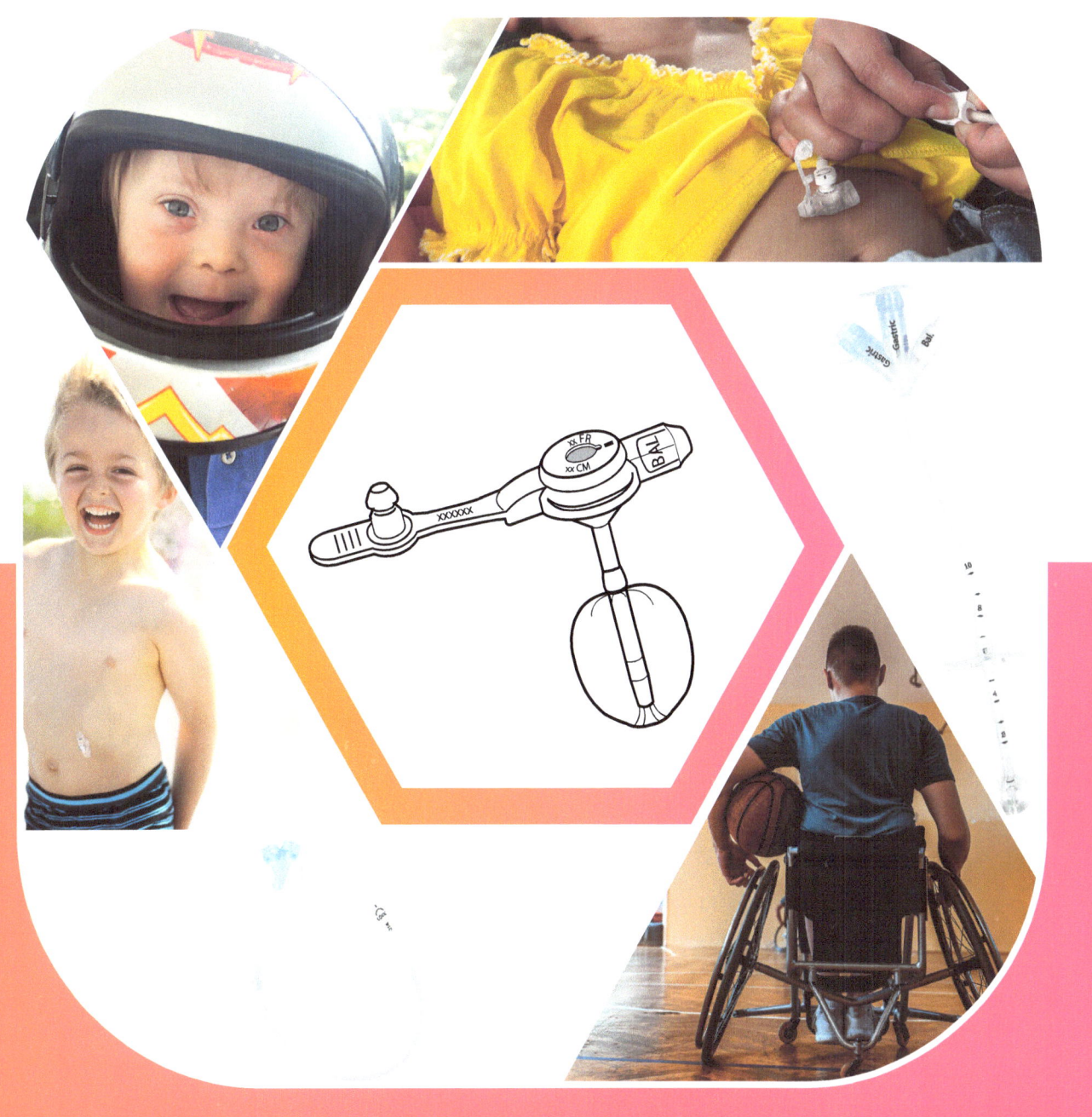

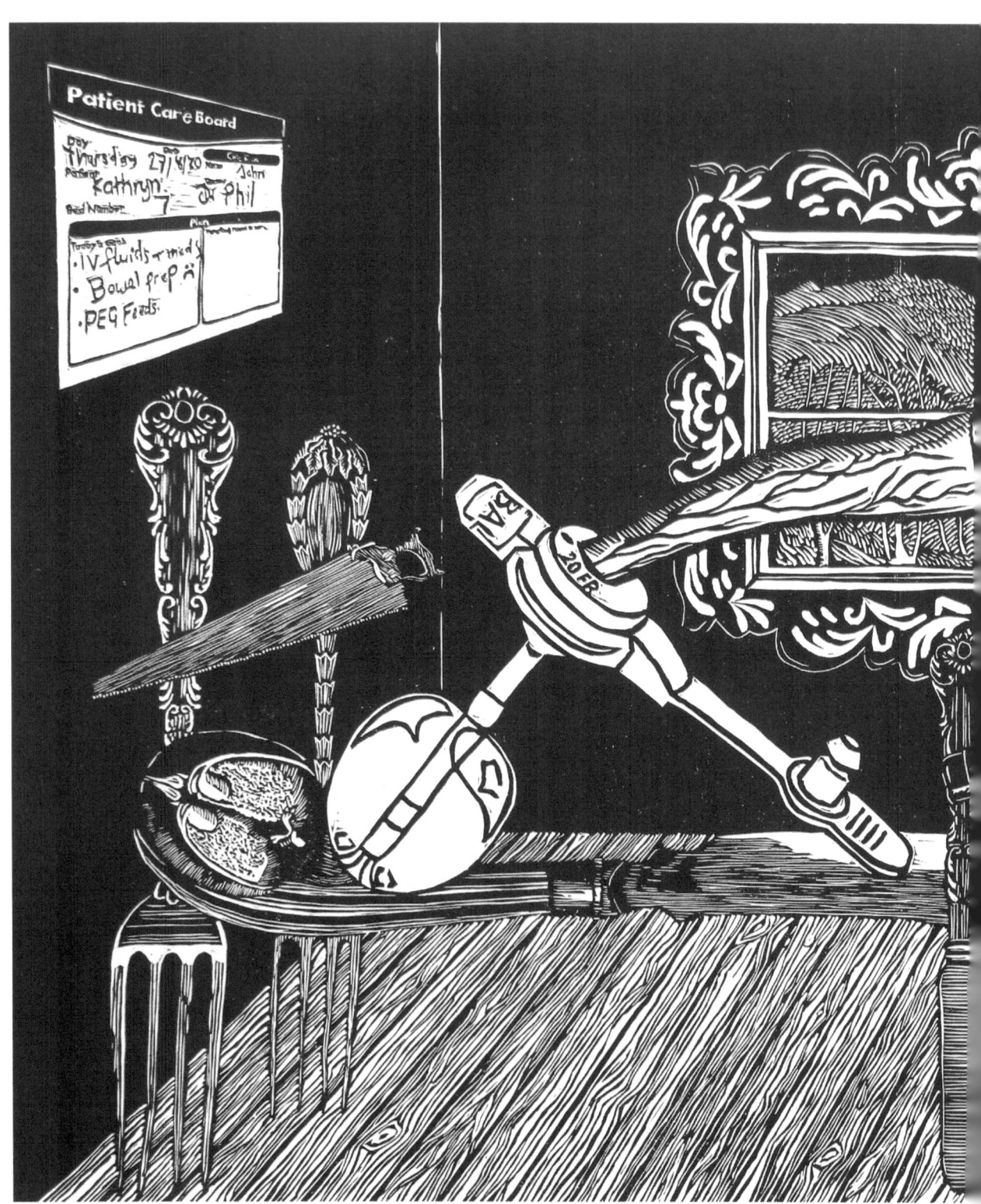

PEG tube in situ, 2021. Linocut print on paper, 56x36cm

/ artist in residence

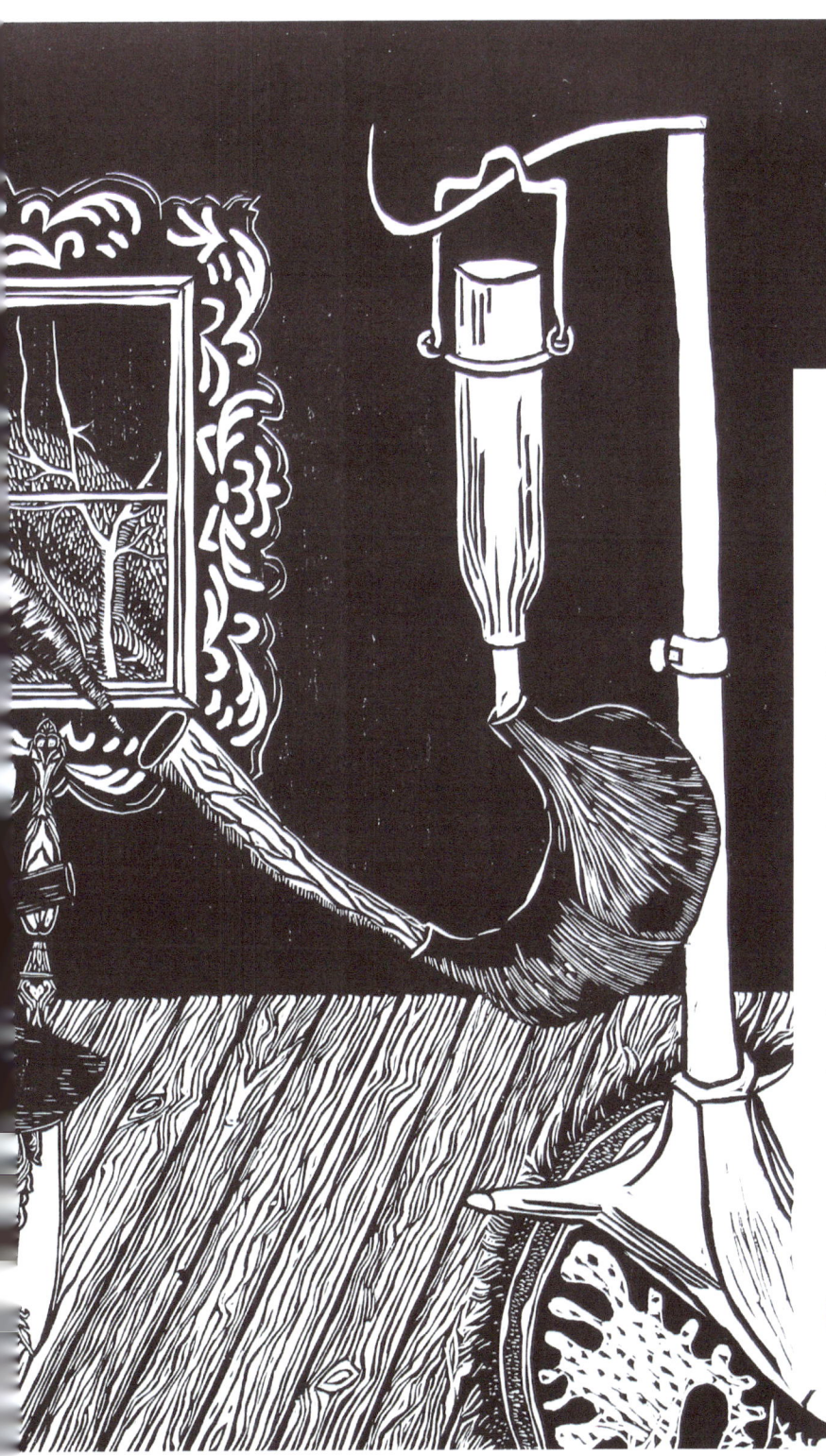

Catch-up with tube-fed artist, Kathryn Lean

'The past year has presented new challenges in life and in tube-feeding for me. I was heavily impacted by the shipping nightmare which found many tube-fed individuals without access to their regular formulas and supplies. It was a challenging time – especially as this occurred at the very beginning of my Master's degree.

'Things are now thankfully back on track and I'm balancing my Master's study in art therapy with my personal art practice. This has been a really interesting process. I'm learning the theory behind my own experiences of using art to express my feelings around my illness and hope to walk alongside others using art therapy in the future.'

Read Kathryn Lean's story in Issue One of The Blend.

Follow her work on Instagram @art.life.Kathy

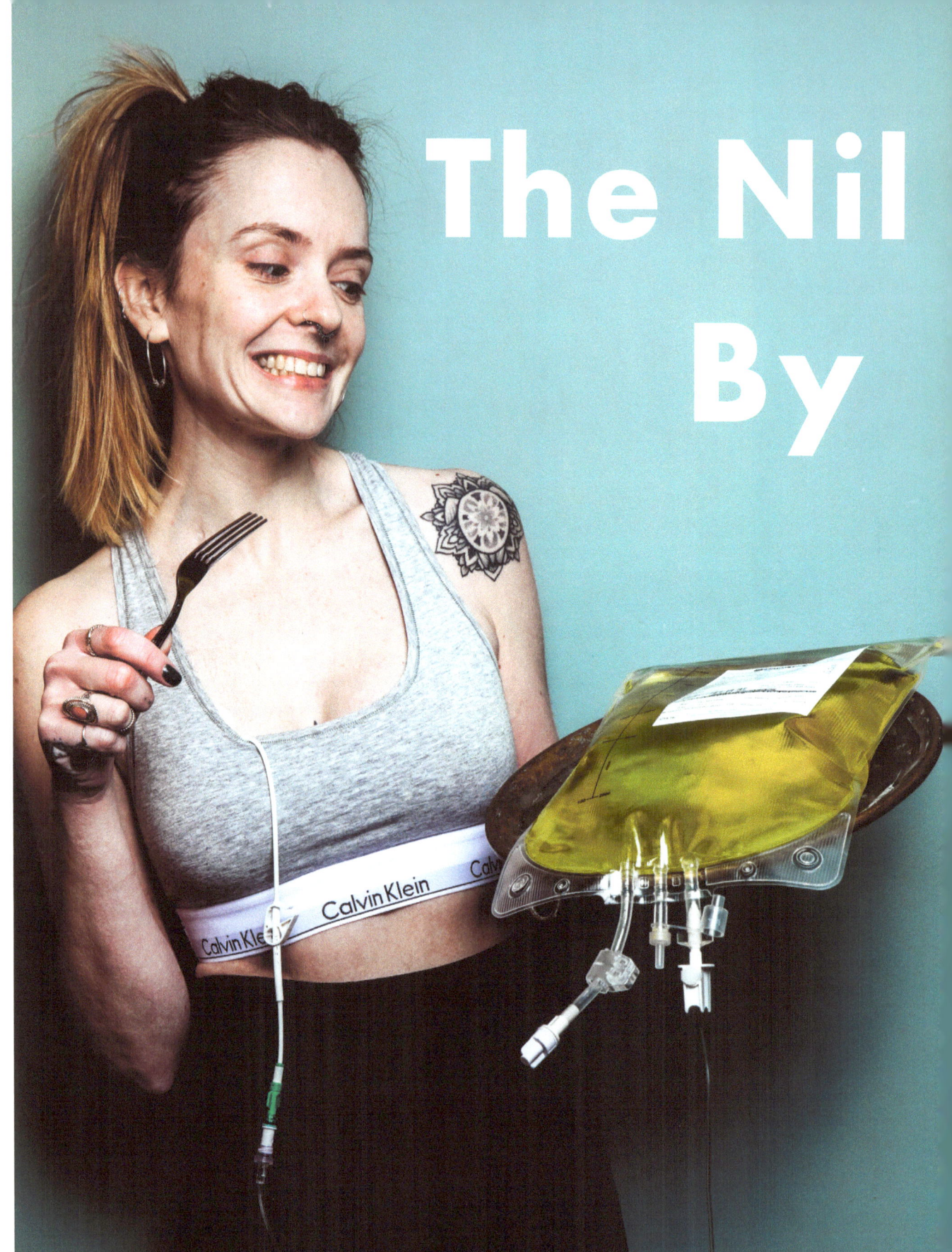

/ cover story

Mouth Foodie

Despite having a digestive system that won't let her eat, Loretta Harmes hasn't lost her appetite for cooking. And since sharing her story and culinary talent with the world, she's been relishing all life has to offer.

Photography: Amy Maidment

As she talks about her wheelchair – a long-resisted development she's recently nestled into – Loretta Harmes exudes her signature, glass-half-full attitude: 'It's giving me freedom and independence, rather than taking it away.'

Speaking from her home in Poole, a coastal town in Dorset, southern England, the 30-year-old sprawls on her bed while pondering the next question: What does it feel like to be fed through your heart?

'I still now – even after being on total parenteral nutrition (TPN) since 2015 – sometimes think all of a sudden, oh, wow, I'm actually fed through there!' she marvels. 'It just hits you sometimes how crazy that is in itself.'

Also known as intravenous or IV nutrition feeding, TPN is a method of feeding liquid nutrients into the body through the veins. Loretta's are delivered through a central venous catheter, called a Hickman line, over 18 hours each day.

'It comes with a mix of emotions,' says Loretta, who hasn't eaten orally for almost eight years. 'It's giving back a lot more than it has taken away and I don't have severe pain now, because my food is going through my bloodstream. So it's a good thing, in that respect.'

Loretta has Ehlers-Danlos syndrome (EDS), a genetic condition causing damage to the connective tissue in the wall of her intestines. She also has gastroparesis, which means her stomach is partially paralysed and can't properly empty itself.

These diagnoses were hard won for Loretta – only coming after years of agonising pain, misdiagnosis and doctors not believing her. She was 12 when her stomach and digestive problems started. At 14 she was diagnosed with irritable bowel syndrome and at 15, disordered eating and digestive issues followed.

In the background of all of this, whenever she could manage it, Loretta took comfort in the very thing that caused her anguish. Food.

'I've had a passion for cooking since I was a little girl,' she says. >>

the blend.

'I just love the hands-on nature of creating things and the freedom it can give you. When I've got ingredients I can do whatever I want with, that really gets my creative juices going.'

Loretta happily divulges her most recent triumph – a convincingly crisp hoisin 'duck' made from mushrooms. 'I couldn't believe it actually worked – and my mum couldn't really tell the difference!' she says.

After years of feeding her family and winning school cooking competitions, Loretta was midway through a top culinary course in London when, at 19, her health took a dramatic dive and she could barely eat or empty her bowels.

One doctor insisted Loretta's weight loss meant the eating disorder she had at 15 must have returned. She spent more than two years in eating disorder units where she was forced to eat and driven to pain and frustration-induced outbursts that saw her sectioned under the Mental Health Act for 18 months.

Loretta had lost all hope and was feeling suicidal when she saw a psychiatrist specialising in gut-brain connection. That psychiatrist told Loretta they'd heard of patients with similar symptoms also not being believed by their medical teams. Emboldened by this discovery, Loretta went to the UK's top Ehlers-Danlos syndrome (EDS) specialist who, in 2015, delivered her long-awaited diagnosis.

> "I just love the hands-on nature of creating things and the freedom it can give you. When I've got ingredients I can do whatever I want with, that really gets my creative juices going."

'I later got tests from my specialist bowel hospital which explained why I was losing weight, in pain and had problems eating,' Loretta recalls. 'After a lengthy hospital stay of trialling ways to eat, I was put on TPN.'

At 23 years old, Loretta's last meal of roast potatoes – cooked to crunchy-and-fluffy perfection – took part in those tests and trials. Does she miss eating orally? Yes, but she feels fortunate not to get cravings for food.

'I was in so much severe agony for years,' says Loretta. 'Food, for me, just equalled pain. It wasn't pleasant. It just filled me with dread.'

Her love of cooking, however, never wavered. And when a BBC interview shared this unlikely chef's story in 2021, the world came to know her as The Nil By Mouth Foodie.

'I can't believe how things escalated from that article,' she says, only days away from launching her business, Nil By Mouth & Co, a 'slow fashion' brand featuring tees and tanks printed with the words: 'Your current situation isn't your final destination.'

Loretta is staunchly philosophical about her own health challenges, but struggles to reconcile with the tragic loss of her younger sister, Abbie.

In 2019, Loretta's mother and Abbie visited Loretta in hospital where she was recovering from sepsis – a common complication for those who feed through TPN. Devastatingly, Abbie died in a car crash on the way home.

'I don't think I'll ever feel peace with that,' says Loretta. 'It's not something that I've really dealt with or processed. Because so much has happened in my life, the way that I've survived is by dissociating or blocking things.' >>

/ cover story

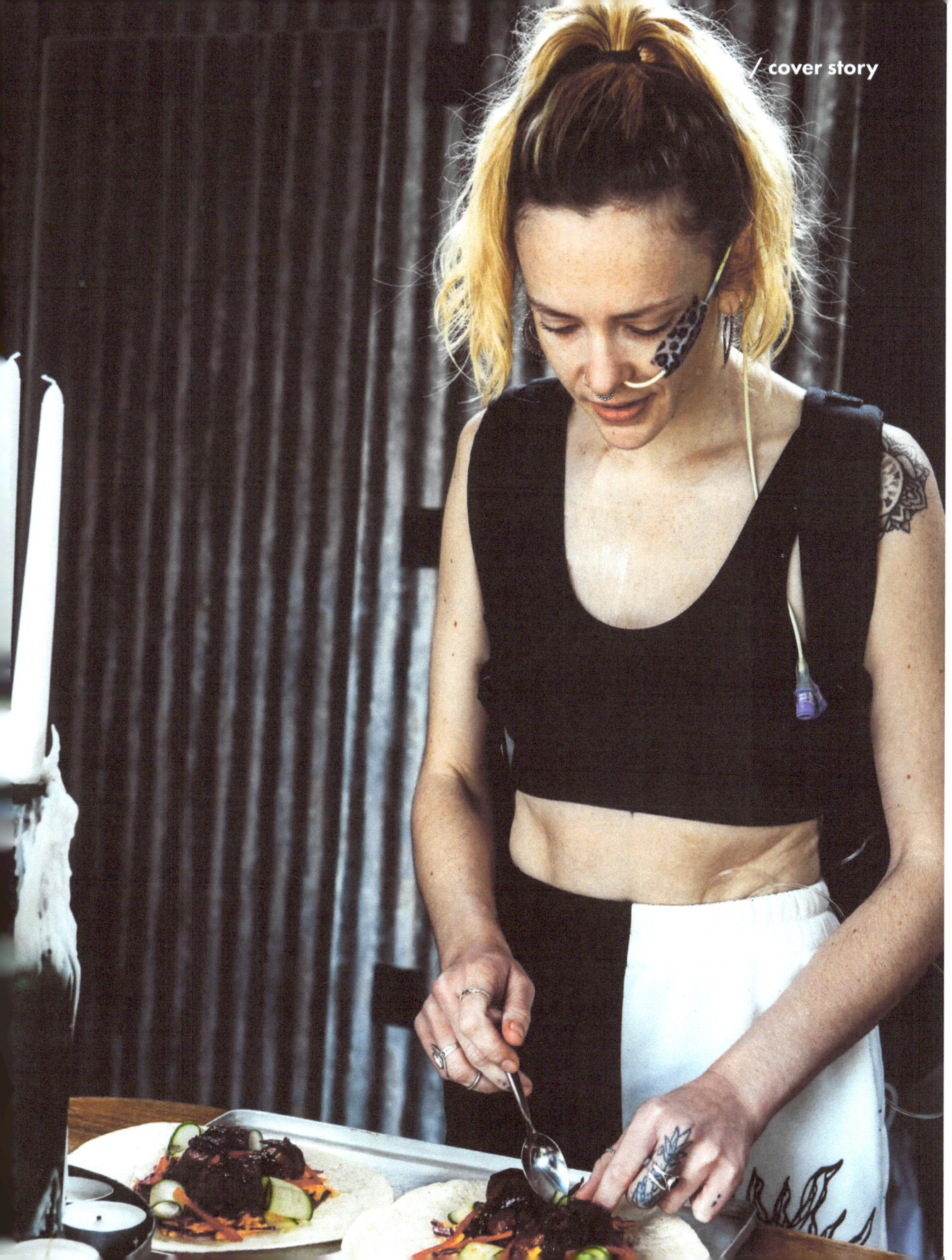

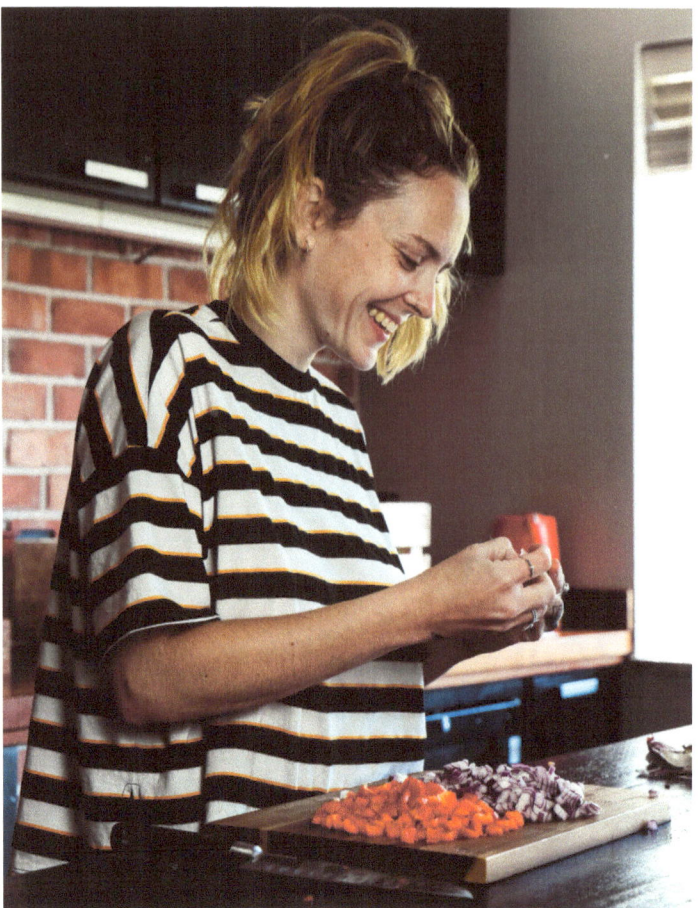

"Something that keeps me going forward is the fact that I need to live for both of us now. That's given me a determination to do as much as I can and try and help as many people as I can. And make the most of being here still."

'But something that keeps me going forward is the fact that I need to live for both of us now. That's given me a determination to do as much as I can and try and help as many people as I can. And make the most of being here still.'

Since the BBC article skyrocketed her profile, Loretta has done a number of pop-up events where she's taken over restaurant and cafe spaces and fed large parties of people. Last August she made 'super salad boxes' for a charity fun day her family held in memory of Abbie, which raised money for Air Ambulance Kent Surrey Sussex.

'We owe them so much for allowing us to say goodbye to her properly,' says Loretta, who filled those boxes with a combination of red-pesto mayo potatoes, roasted balsamic vegetables and tahini dressed lettuce with seasoned crunchy chickpeas. 'I went for salads because a lot of people came – and I didn't want to be on a stool cooking all day.'

Loretta's 'whizzy' stool – like her wheelchair – is one of her many workarounds for getting about with greater ease. She uses tubie clips to keep her line secure, a portable car fridge to keep her formula cold, and a backpack to carry her feed bag wherever she goes.

'It's actually a nappy bag,' she says. 'They're amazing for feeding stuff because they've got so many compartments. You can put all of your medications and little nifty bits in there that you need – and they tend to be waterproof. I also found a wheelie trolly that I can put my bag on. So if it's too heavy on my back, I can put my bag on there and go about my business.'

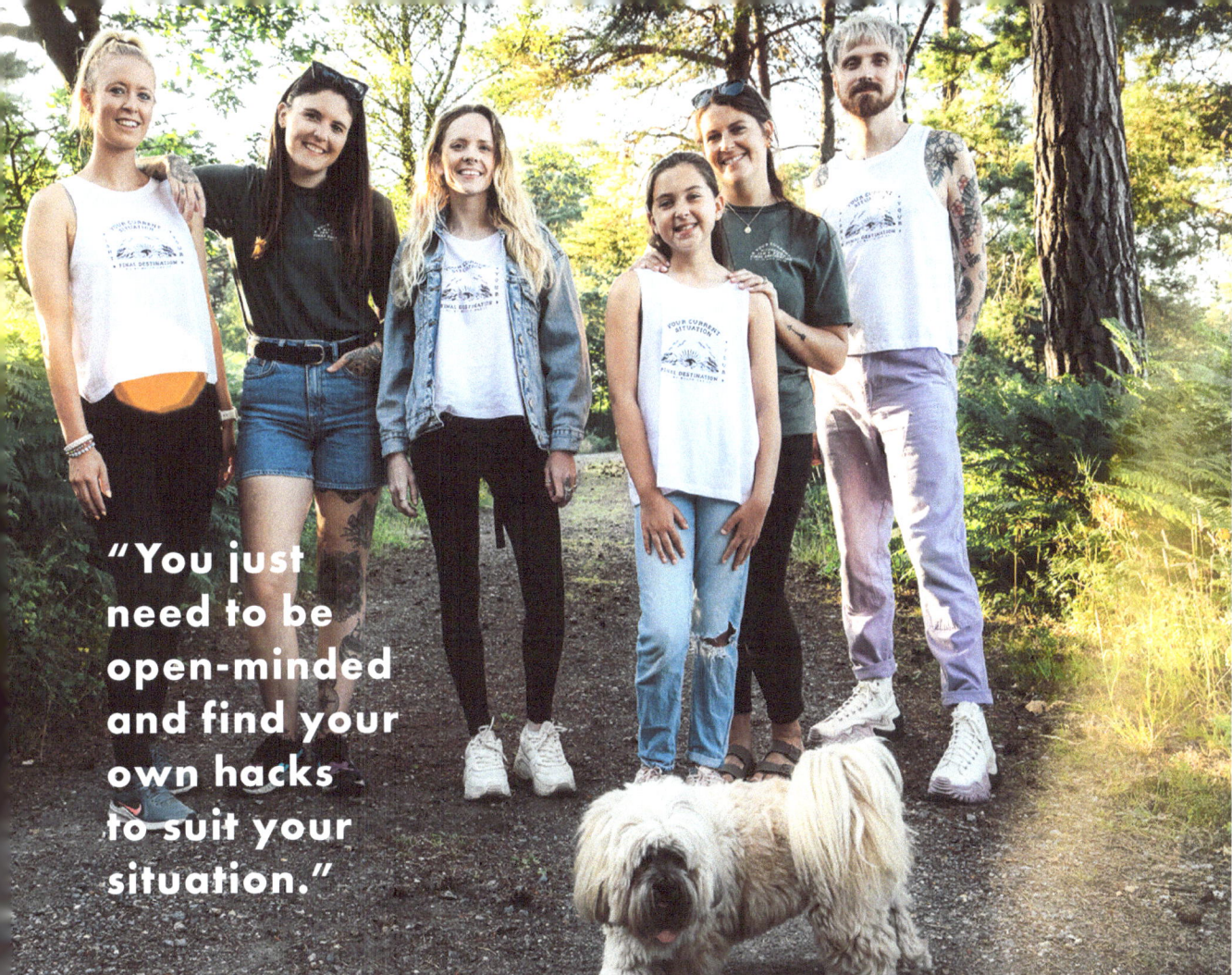

"You just need to be open-minded and find your own hacks to suit your situation."

In addition to her Hickman line for TPN, Loretta now has a jejunal tube. Or as she calls it, 'Jeff'.

In an especially cunning fix, Loretta has found a way to take Jeff into a jacuzzi – usually a big no-no for anyone with a G or J-tube. She manages this by squeezing Jeff into a 'swimming dressing' designed for her Hickman line. 'For those who can't get that type of dressing, stoma bags would 100 per cent do the job,' she says.

When Loretta hits an obstacle, she finds a way around it – and says it tends to be mindsets, rather than medical devices, that hold people back.

'Doctors don't always make it sound as though you can live a fulfilled, normal life,' she says. 'They can be very medically oriented because they're not living it – they're only seeing tube-feeding in a hospital environment. So it took me some time to try and rewire that belief. You just need to be open-minded and find your own hacks to suit your situation.'

Oral eating will never be an option for Loretta – but bowel feeding could be. Back when she started TPN, she also tried feeding through a nasojejunal (NJ) tube. This didn't last long, 'because my bowel was in such a bad state at that point'. She tried more NJs for getting medication down, but they all failed.

'I'm fully accepting of TPN now but at the same time, there's always anxiety and worry because it's a very extreme way of feeding with severe complications,' says Loretta. 'It only takes a small speck of dust in the line to cause sepsis – which I've had nine times. When sepsis happens you can't feed through your line because it's infected, and you can't put another line in because your blood's contaminated. You have to starve that bacteria – which means starving me.'

During one of those nine bouts of sepsis, Loretta lived on nothing more than a saline drip for 16 days. 'If you happen to get in one of those situations you feel out of control, because you can't do anything,' she says. >>

the blend. 71

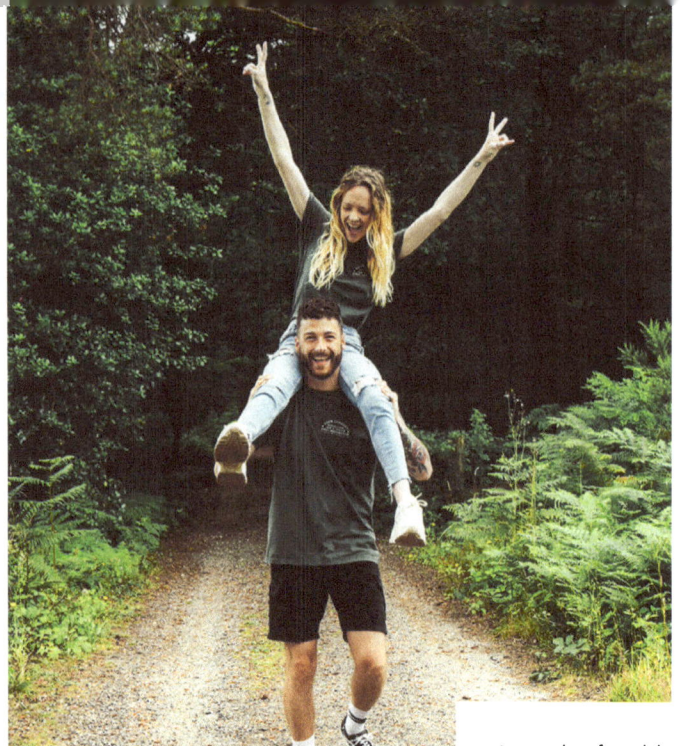

"You can still have a really good quality of life despite the tubes, despite medical devices, despite the diagnosis. They don't define you."

'Last year I pleaded with my consultant to give an NJ just one more try, because my bowel has settled and rested. To my surprise – and everyone else's – I got on OK with taking medications through it, to the point where we could change to a jejunostomy (J) tube. Whether or not I come off of TPN completely, it will still be good to be able to get whatever I can get down the J-tube. That's an achievement in itself.'

The standard elemental and semi-elemental formulas designed for bowel feeding aren't sitting well with Loretta, so she's looking into making her own. Whenever she can find time, that is.

Currently developing recipes and doing food styling for brands, Loretta has been approached by several agencies eager to help her publish a memoir. 'Something on TV could be happening as well,' she hints. 'There are many eggs in the basket.'

They say you should never trust a chef who doesn't eat their own food, but Loretta has found that once taste leaves the building, other senses come to the party.

'My sense of smell has heightened so much since not eating – which I guess is my body's natural response of trying to balance things out. I always think about a recipe before I cook it and while I'm cooking I kind of just know how to balance the flavours. It's like someone's in my ear. I get other people to taste my food and most of the time I'm not far off. Things might just need a bit of tweaking.'

When she's not cooking, Loretta goes to restaurants and bars with her family, partner and friends. 'If we go out I'll always ask, is there a pool table? It's about finding things I can enjoy when food is involved,' she says.

Loretta lives with housemate Amy Maidment, a photographer who's captured much of Loretta's work since she left her family home in Sussex.

'I moved here with just a food blog and when the article came out, it gave me an opportunity to create more of a life and share my experiences as well, which was really important for me because I was unheard for so long,' says Loretta.

'I want to keep sharing and help others with what I've learnt over my years of being tube-fed.'

What message does she have for people who are new to this space?

'You can still have a really good quality of life despite the tubes, despite medical devices, despite the diagnosis. They don't define you. It's a really hard adjustment and it will take time to accept, but know that it does get easier. This thing is giving you your life back. It's special and you just need to get adventurous in how you go about things.'

Find Loretta's roasted coconutty butternut squash soup recipe on page 126.

 thenilbymouthfoodie.com
@the.nil.by.mouth.foodie
Nil By Mouth & Co

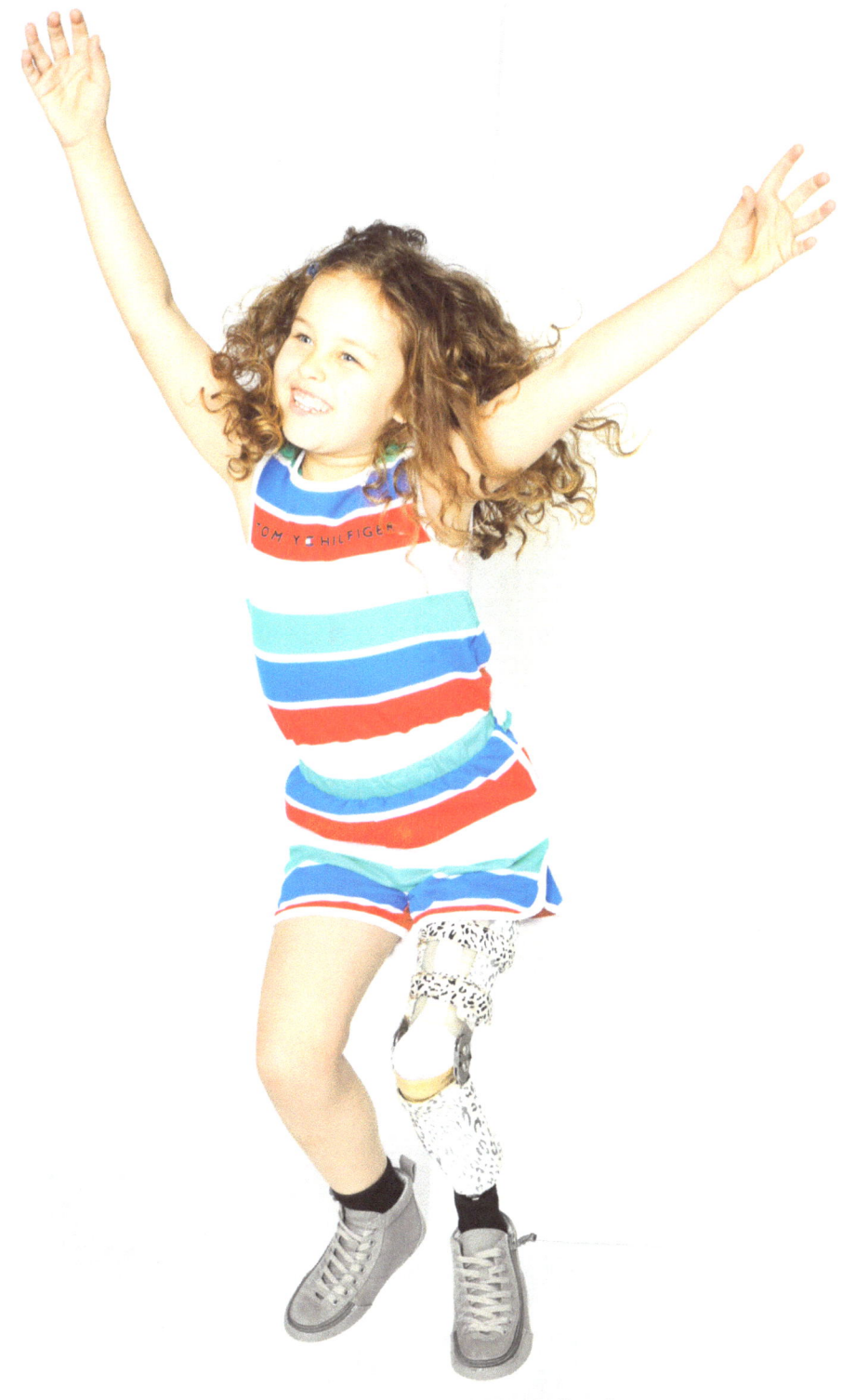

Fashion, Footwear and Lifestyle for All

EVERYHUMAN

Read us online:

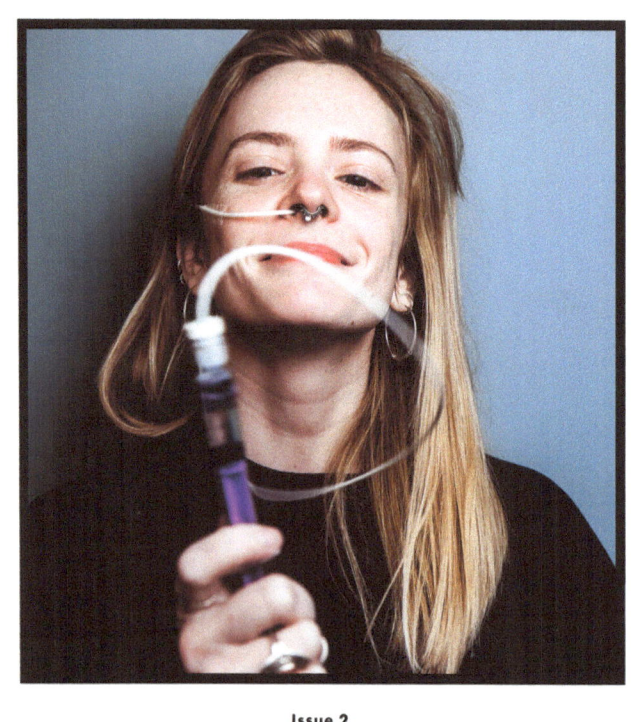

theblendmag.com

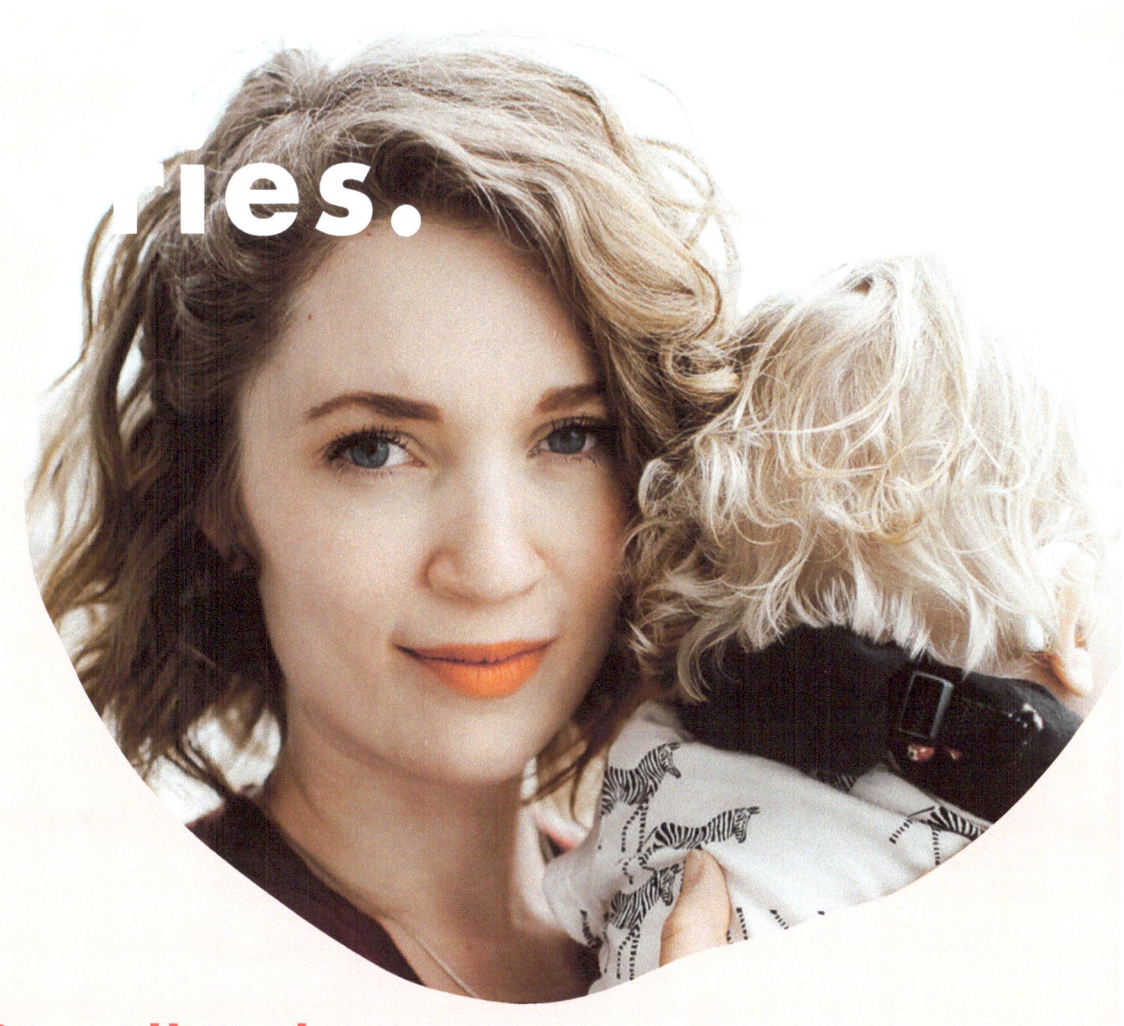

+ Nina Alhambra

+ Eliana Joseph

+ Madeline Cheney

+ Brana Gadsby & Ross Worth

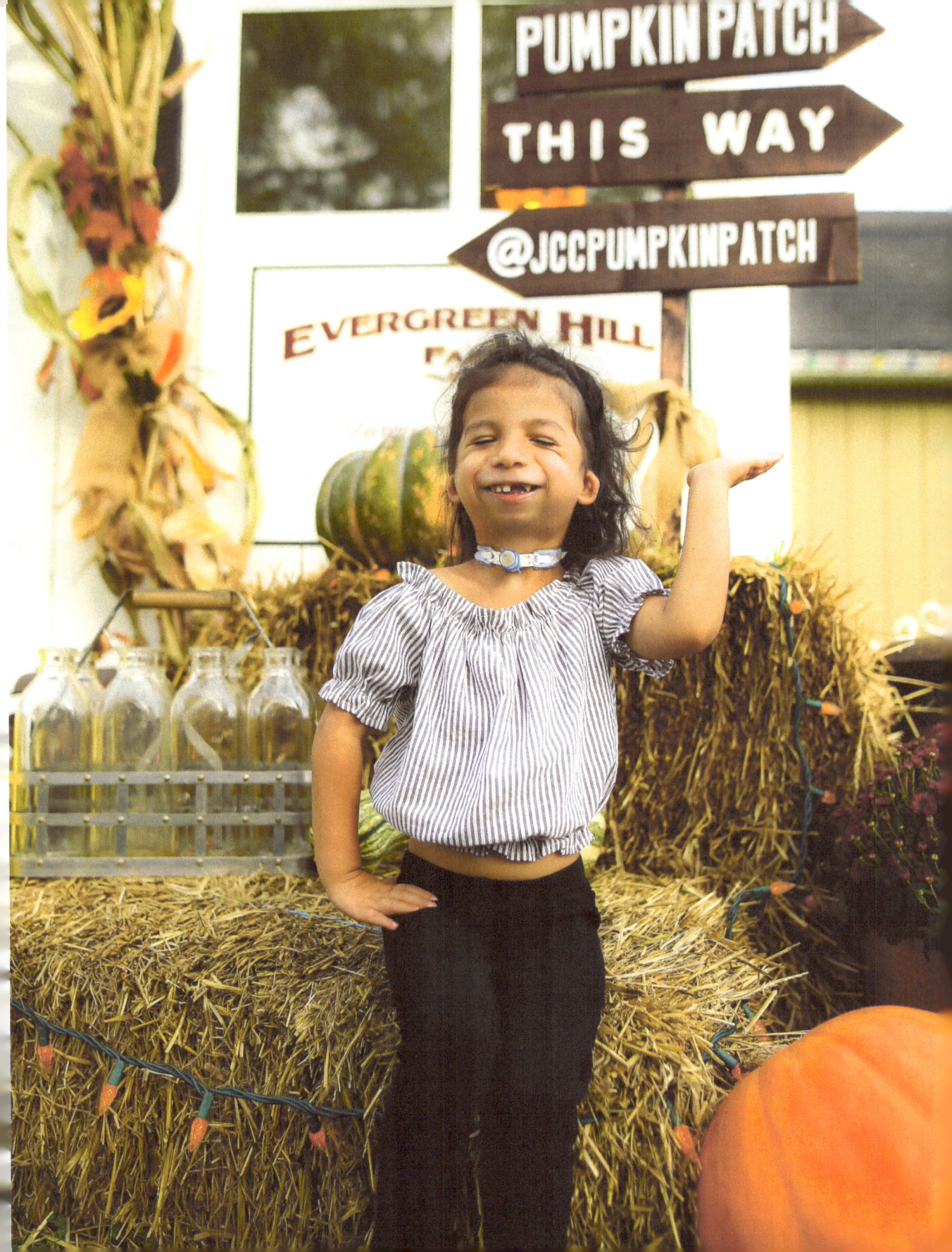

/ parent stories

Tubie truths

They can't always eat when they're hungry, the number on the scale doesn't tell the full picture and, no matter what, things will be OK. These and other hard-earned lessons spill freely from Toronto-based Nina Alhambra, whose four-year-old daughter has transitioned off her G-tube.

How did tube-feeding come into your life? My daughter, Emily, was born with Treacher Collins syndrome and the characteristics that come with that, like a cleft palate and recessed jaw, made it very difficult to eat. She started on a nasogastric (NG) tube, which the doctors sold to us as 'not permanent'.

Emily also drank from a specialised bottle that worked with her cleft palate at the time. There was hope that she'd be able to eat orally, but we were far from it. Emily hated the NG tube. She was pulling it out numerous times a day.

How did you deal with that? Did you learn how to put the tube in yourself, or were you in and out of hospital? The medical team taught us how to place it. Mind you, it was awful. Emily was in the hospital for the first two months of her life. My husband worked for long periods, so I was by myself. Having to insert that tube several times a day on my own was traumatising for both me and Emily. I was also completely obsessed with how much she was eating.

My sister, who has three children of her own, said, 'if she's taking a bottle and she doesn't finish it, maybe she's full'. I was really confused because everyone kept saying, 'if she's hungry, she's going to eat'. But it was exhausting for her to eat.

Emily was born at a good weight but she declined so quickly. The skin was hanging off her bones. Her head looked so much bigger than her body and the amount of weight she was losing was really scary.

I was feeding her my breast milk through the NG tube and with the specialised bottle and she just kept throwing up. I thought, is it my breast milk? Am I the reason why she's not gaining weight? >>

the blend.

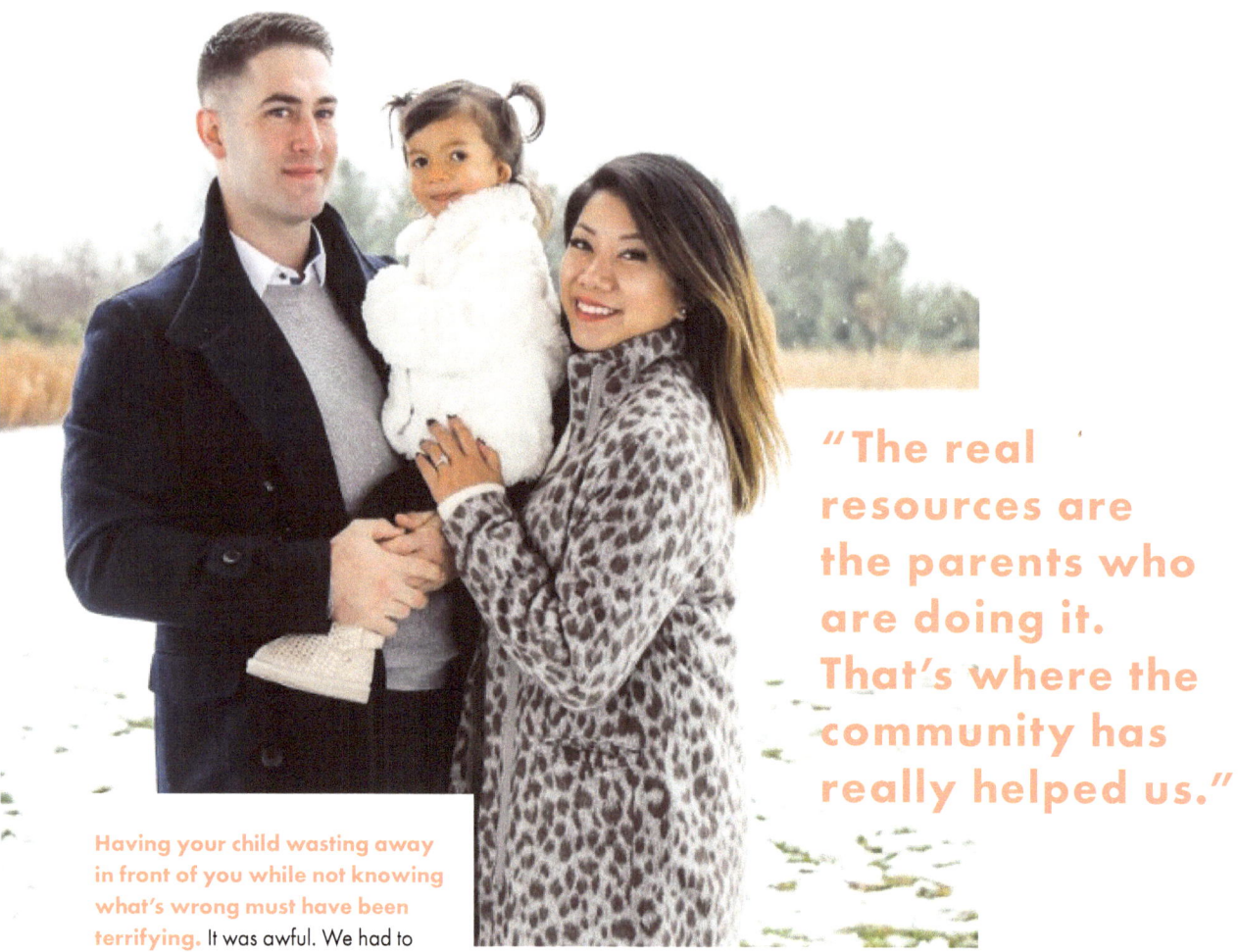

"The real resources are the parents who are doing it. That's where the community has really helped us."

Having your child wasting away in front of you while not knowing what's wrong must have been terrifying. It was awful. We had to go to the doctor's office once a week to weigh her. I remember holding my breath every time and they'd say, 'she lost weight again'. We had to get readmitted to the hospital because she was showing signs of dehydration.

We talked about the gastrostomy (G) tube at this point and for us it was really scary because she'd already been through a couple of major surgeries. Did she really need another one? And another hole in her body? She already has a tracheostomy tube.

Now in hindsight, I wish we had the G-tube from the beginning to avoid all of the hardships that came with the NG tube. But at the time it felt like we were taking a huge step backwards.

What happened once the G-tube went in? Emily's recovery was very quick, but then there were a ton of other complications that came after that. We were using a feeding pump and we started fortifying my breast milk – adding some formula to help her gain weight. Every single feed, she was still projectile vomiting.

We'd tried everything to prevent it, like feeding her in an upright position and elevating her bed. We were venting her as well and it just wasn't working. We went to only formula because I was so stressed out that I couldn't produce breast milk anymore. Even still, the vomiting just continued.

It wasn't until she was six months old that I started hearing about blended feeds. I tried talking to my medical team about switching her and they were not supportive. They put her on medication to help with her reflux, but she was still vomiting every day.

Thankfully, I had a social worker and she made me feel really validated in my concerns. Using her connections she found another mum whose daughter was a couple of months older than Emily and had switched to a full blended diet.

My social worker said, 'let me connect you to this mum and you guys can talk it out'. And we did. As wonderful as it is to meet people through social

/ **parent stories**

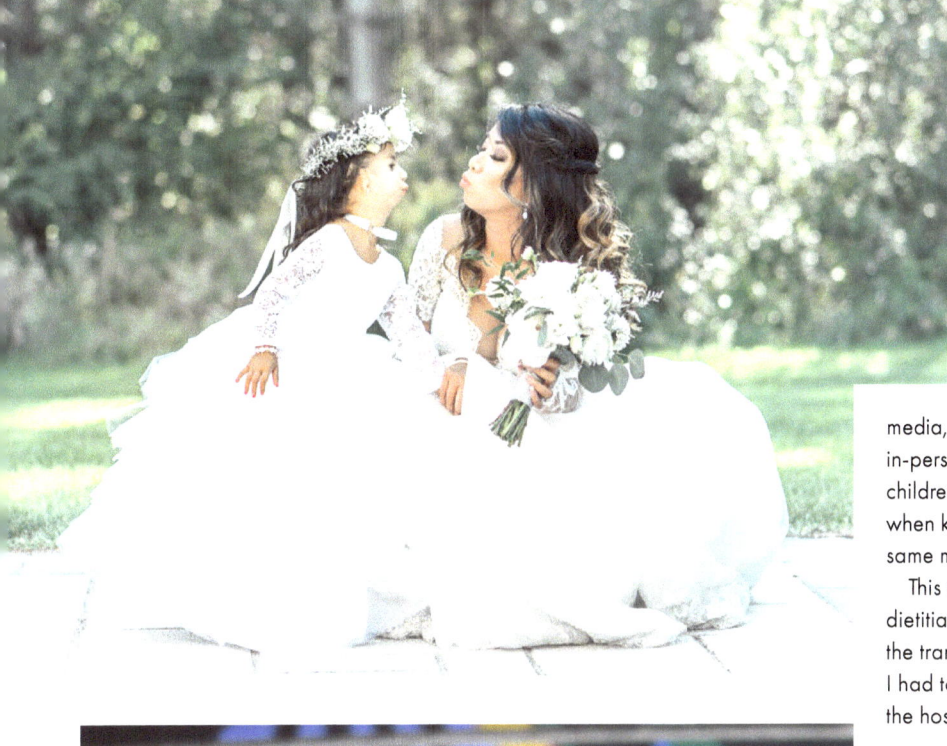

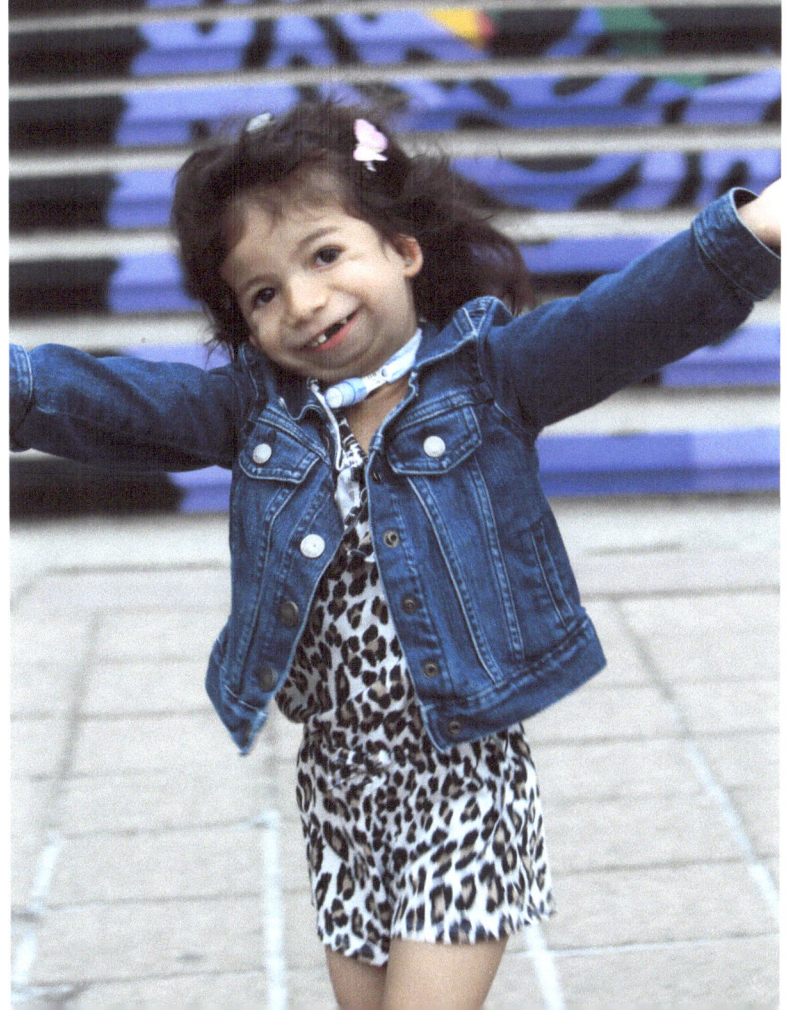

media, there's just something about that in-person connection and having your children meet. It's always really cool when kids discover that they have the same medical accessories.

This mum referred me to a wonderful dietitian who supported us in making the transition to blends. It's something I had to hide from my medical team at the hospital.

Because you were breaking the rules, right? Yes! I always felt like we had to ask for permission or get approval from someone who knew what the right answer was. And then I learnt that they were comparing Emily to a textbook where they got their information. The real resources are the parents who are doing it. That's where the community has really helped us.

Our dietitian helped me slowly introduce blends into Emily's formula, one ingredient at a time, and we quickly saw a decline in her vomiting. I was terrified to switch to syringe feeding, but once I did, we never went back to our feeding pump.

Then I started seeing dietitian Claire Kariya's blend recipes on Instagram. I started really simple and blended Emily some toast with peanut butter and jam with milk. It felt so special to be able to do that. To not be so strict about having specific ingredients and food groups. To just pick meals that I know my nieces and nephews were having and feed her that way. >>

the blend. 79

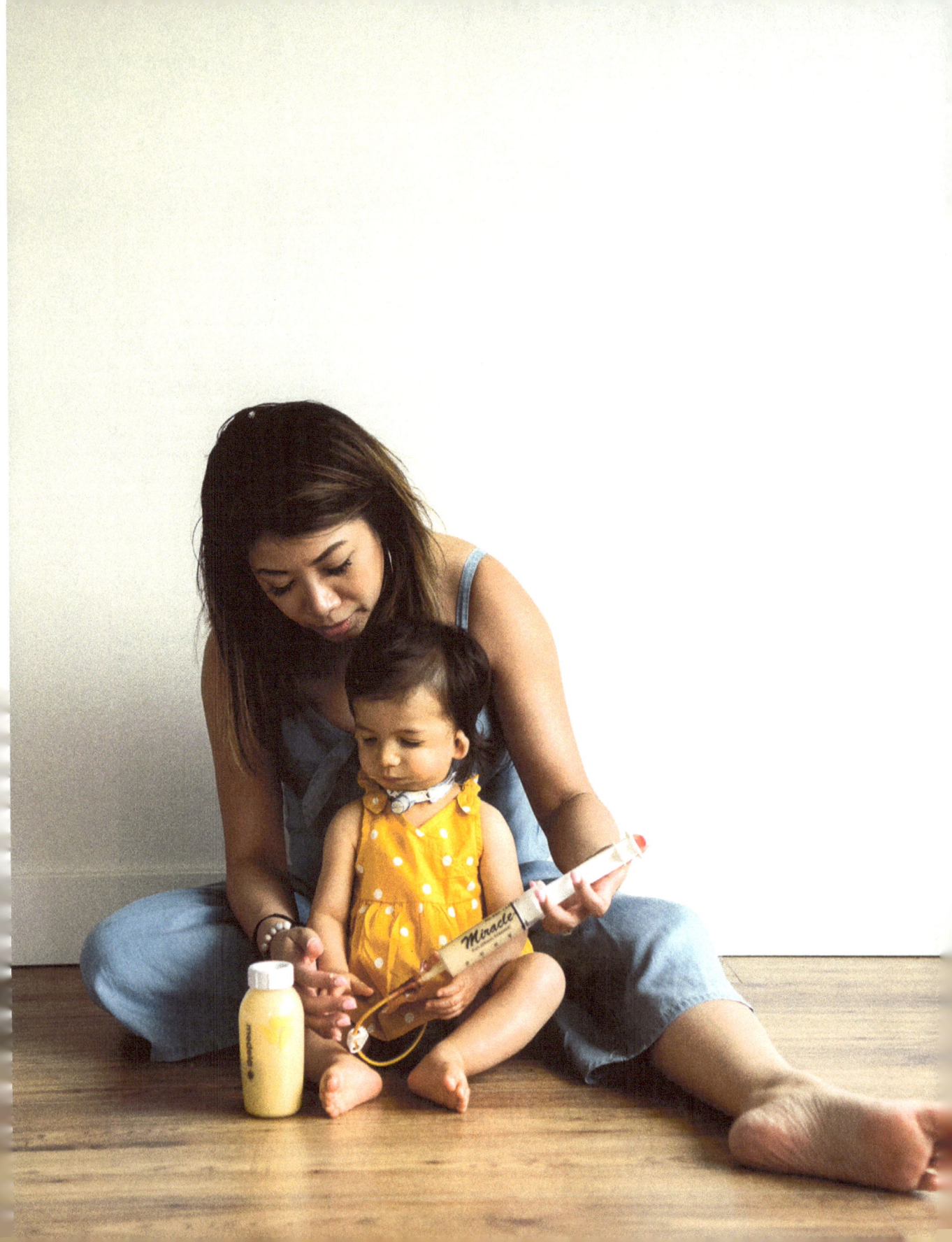

/ parent stories

I get that – and love nothing more than blending up a piece of cake for Arlo when we're celebrating. You say Emily's vomiting decreased with the blends, what happened with her weight?
That's still something I'm dealing with. Her medical team stresses me out about it, because they weigh her at each appointment. Their obsession with her weight gave me an obsession with her weight. The last in-person appointment we had with them was around two years ago now and she'd lost weight. At this point we'd weaned her off most of her tube feeds. Her cleft palate was repaired, which helped with her oral eating.

The doctors couldn't understand her weight loss because her colour looked good. She was communicating really well, she was bright and expressive. She didn't match that number on the scale. They were questioning it to the point that they were weighing themselves to make sure the scale wasn't broken. They allocated us a dietitian who would come and see us every week and weigh her. They said that if she didn't start gaining, we'd have to go back to the tube-feeds.

Thankfully, that dietitian was very supportive of us and our choices. I told him that we might have to start tube-feeding again and he said, 'no, we will modify what she's eating'. We're not moving backwards, is what he said. That's not what we're going to do.

Nowadays I track Emily's growth by how her clothes fit. Eventually I just told myself, don't weigh her anymore. I still think about it a lot, but I don't put her on the scale anymore.

That sounds like some solid sanity-preservation right there. So Emily is feeding orally now?
She is. We still have to make some adjustments – like cutting her food up really small – and she does take a long time to eat. But from the get-go, she has had a huge interest in eating. We do have the G-tube still placed for medication and vitamins. And if ever we're thinking she didn't eat enough and we need to supplement for that day, especially if she's sick, we'll use it as well. I'm kind of scared of the day coming when our team says she can get rid of it.

By the time this magazine comes out you'll have welcomed your second child. How are you feeling about heading back into newborn territory? Kind of terrified. I don't know if our next child is going to have any medical needs, but in any case, I won't know how to navigate being a new mum again because our first experience was so different.

Having said that, I can take what we've learnt over these last few years and I'll know that everything will be OK. I just wish that I could go back in time and tell new-mum me that everything is going to work out, one way or another. It's still really, really hard, but we're happy. Emily's happy.

A little (and very exciting) update from Nina since she was interviewed for this story: 'Emily's feeding tube broke and we didn't have a spare so we made the decision to leave it out. Her doctor had been so happy with her progress that we felt comfortable making this decision. So far, she's been doing well without it. And we had a baby boy!'

 @neens.nicole

> "I just wish that I could go back in time and tell new-mum me that everything is going to work out, one way or another. It's still really, really hard, but we're happy. Emily's happy."

the blend. 81

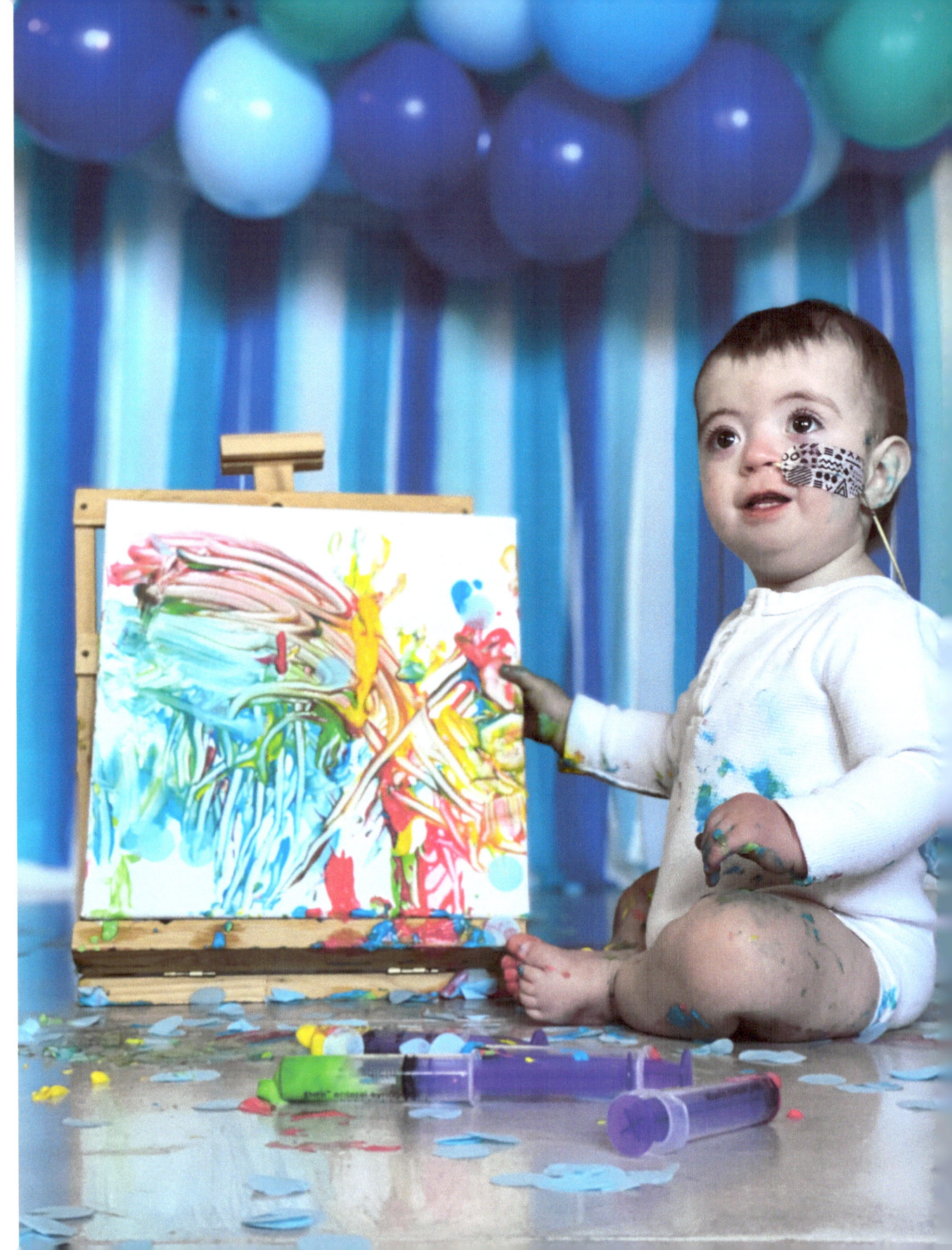

/ parent stories

Smashing it

Tube-feeding came as a shock to Eliana Joseph when her baby son, Luke, entered the world on a wave of uncertainties. But it didn't take this unexpected advocate long to find her groove. Nowadays Luke is having his cake and (working on) eating it too.

You celebrated Luke's first birthday with your own version of a 'cake smash' photo shoot. Cheers to that! Luke had been nil-by-mouth for the majority of his life and we'd only just got the OK for him to have thickened purees safely, so I wanted to do something really special for him with a tubie twist. I popped up a post asking for ideas on the Feeding Tube Australia Facebook group and lots of people came back to me.

One woman suggested putting dyed yoghurt in Luke's syringes – a great idea, because he likes to play with his syringes, too. Then I got a canvas and thought, we'll do some painting and make it messy and he can just get it everywhere. I don't care and it'll look great!

I love how you make sure Luke doesn't miss out on the fun stuff, even if it means getting creative or, I'm guessing, lugging around a bunch of tube-feeding kit. Absolutely. I'll meet up with some friends for a walk and they'll see what I've got in my pram and actually apologise. Like, 'I'm so sorry that we asked you'. And I'm like, why? If you don't ask me, what am I going to do, stay at home all day? No thanks.

How did tube-feeding first come into your life? It was quite a rude shock. I had my daughter, Leah, four years before Luke was born and she was completely fine. My birth with her was quite traumatic, however, so my biggest fear about having another one was having to go through the birth. The birth went great but as soon as he came out, he couldn't breathe properly and that was where it all started.

Luke started to turn blue and then they took him off to the special care unit. They kept saying that they thought he had some kind of obstruction but they didn't know what was going on. When he was first born they did try to put him on the boob and the poor thing just couldn't even attempt it. He was tube-fed from the get-go and his NG (nasogastric) tube became a regular fixture.

Did you get an explanation as to why there were troubles? The medical team discovered Luke has a floppy epiglottis which we were told would improve – and I believe it has, to a degree. >>

the blend.

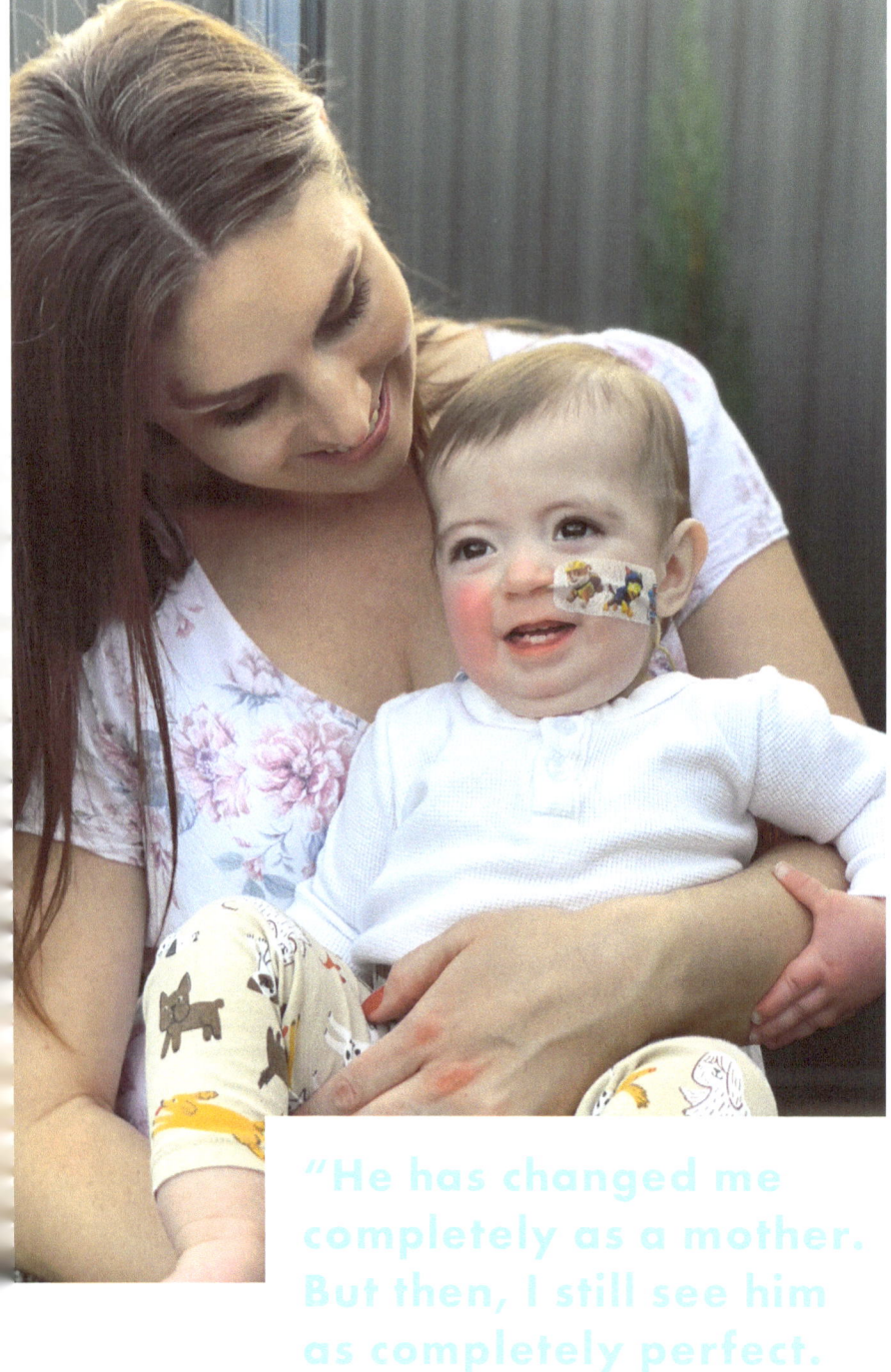

"He has changed me completely as a mother. But then, I still see him as completely perfect. At the start I was very much thinking, when is the tube going?"

Later on we found out he couldn't actually swallow. I thought he was going well with taking a bottle, but his first swallow study showed he was actually silently aspirating on everything.

That was a huge, upsetting shock because I thought he just needed a bit of practice on the bottle and then we could get rid of the tube and it would all be OK. But as hard as that moment was, it was actually a really good turning point for me. I accepted the tube. I accepted that it's here and that it's here to stay. That's just the way it's going to be and that's OK.

Now we finally have a diagnosis for Luke – he has a genetic muscular condition affecting the TNNC2 gene. There are only five other people in the world who have it, Luke now being the sixth. There's not a whole lot of information on it yet so we don't know too much, but we're so relieved to have an answer.

You're pretty new to this and seem to have really found your stride. You've even kept your business going – The Handmade Baby Boutique. Am I right in thinking that, prior to Luke coming along, this only catered to your typical sort of parenthood experience? Yes. So I'm a primary school teacher originally. When I had Leah I didn't want to go back to work – I wanted to be at home with her – but I needed something else, so I created the boutique. I started off by making milestone cards that described what you go through in your first year with your 'normal' kid.

/ parent stories

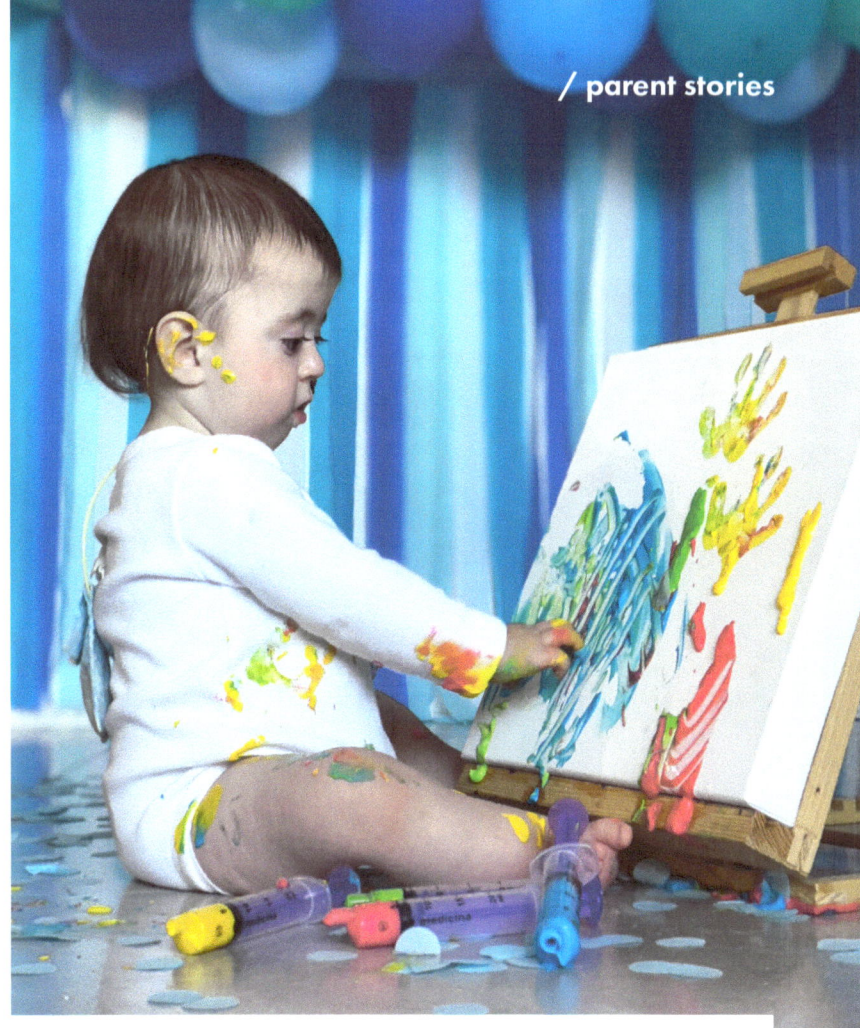

It's interesting now, because I've been using a set with Luke and I'm thinking, we haven't used that one, that one or that one. That one will come later and that's OK. I made some tubie milestone cards with the help of some of the mums in the Feeding Tube Australia Facebook group and it's been nice to be able to have a little pack just for Luke, to celebrate him.

I bet nowadays you look at typical milestones differently. I was scrolling through your Instagram account and found an old picture of a milestone card that says 'perfection' on it. How has your experience with Luke changed your view on parenthood? He has changed me completely as a mother. But then, I still see him as completely perfect. At the start I was very much thinking, when is the tube going? When are we not doing this anymore? When is he going to be like Leah was? But now I know he's not and I wouldn't change him. I wouldn't. And he has changed me so much.

I'm a very quiet person and avoid confrontation at all costs, but there was a point where we weren't being heard by some of Luke's specialists. And I told them off. It was such a huge thing for me – completely out of my comfort zone – but I thought, if I'm not going to do it, no one's going to do it for him. He's taught me to stand up, have some guts and say something.

You become an advocate, don't you? You don't even know you have that in you and then suddenly, bam! And you're raising awareness of tube-feeding with your social following, too. A lot of people have said it's nice for them to read what I've been posting because it makes them feel less alone. That gives me a lot of joy and a lot of comfort, knowing that I can help someone else, too. And I've actually made a really good friend through Instagram, who lives in Adelaide. I've never met her in person but we chat almost every day. Her little boy is a couple of months older than Luke and they have so much in common.

How have you looked after yourself through all of this – have you done any therapy? It's funny actually because with my first I had a lot of postnatal anxiety. I was really concerned that this was going to come up again with Luke but I've handled it all quite well. My psychologist is probably wondering how I went, and I'd have a story to tell her!

I've not gone back to therapy, but one thing I did start trying recently is going to a meditation class and I think it's helped me. I also go to the gym every day. The kids go to the creche, I've got my friends there, we chat and have coffee afterwards. I keep doing that – that's my normality.

the blend.

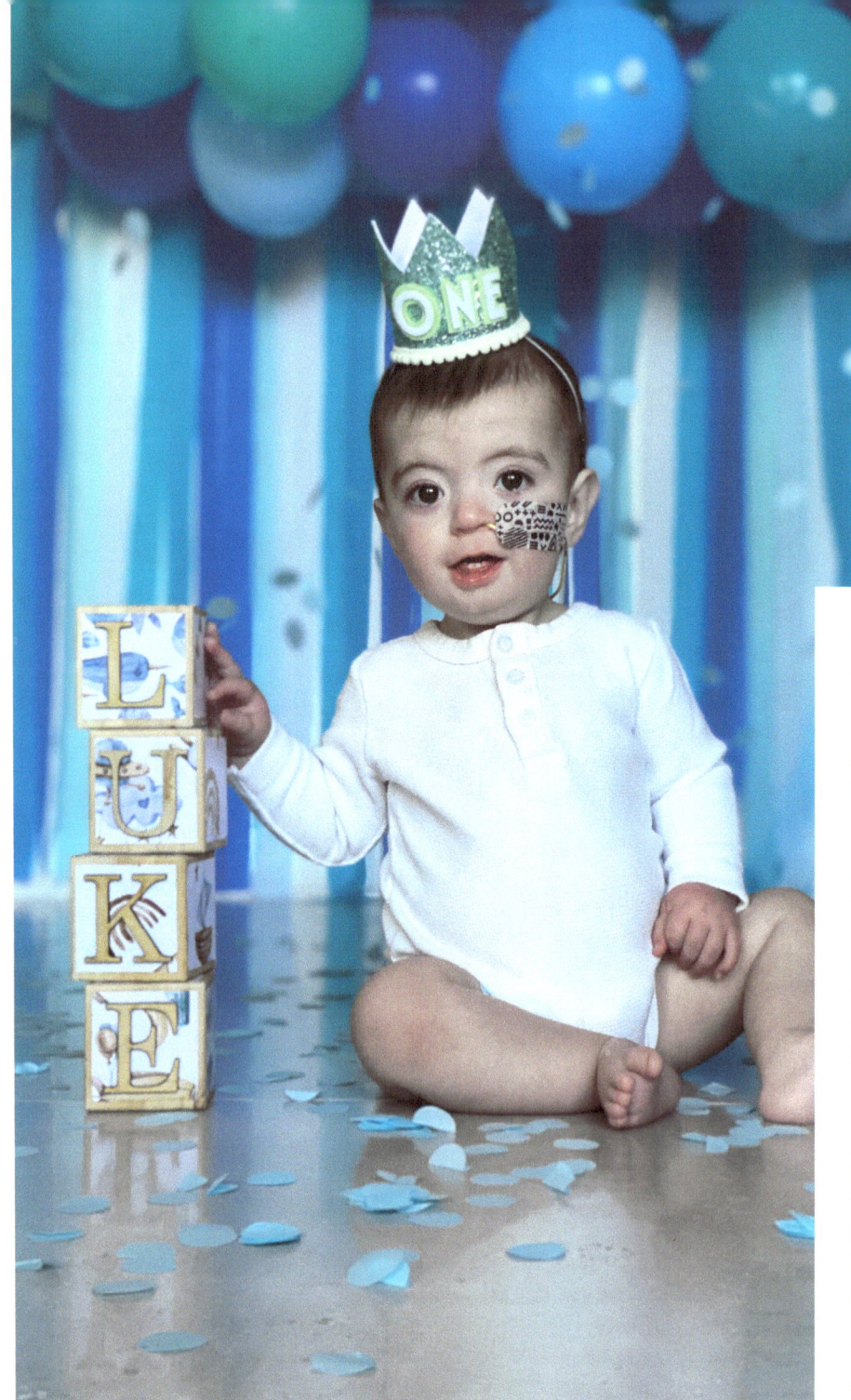

Are they cool with Luke's tube at the creche? They are – and they don't need to feed him. They were very nervous at first because they didn't know what it was, so I showed them the NG tube, hooked the feed up and explained that it goes all the way to his stomach. They were like, all the way? And I was like, yeah, there's a good 28cm worth of tube there!

Luke recently transitioned to a G-tube, what's that been like? Overall, the transition has gone smoothly but surgery day was really tough. The procedure itself went well but was traumatising for both Luke and myself. As soon as we arrived at the hospital Luke knew something was up. He snuggled into me and I cuddled him back, holding his hand, kissing his forehead and telling him how brave he was and that it would all be OK. I hated this for him and my anxiety had been running high for weeks, but I needed to hold it together and stay strong for him.

The doctors had trouble getting him to sleep and it just went on and on. I was warned it would be hard to see but thought 'it's all good, I've got this', but I didn't have anything. It became too much

/ parent stories

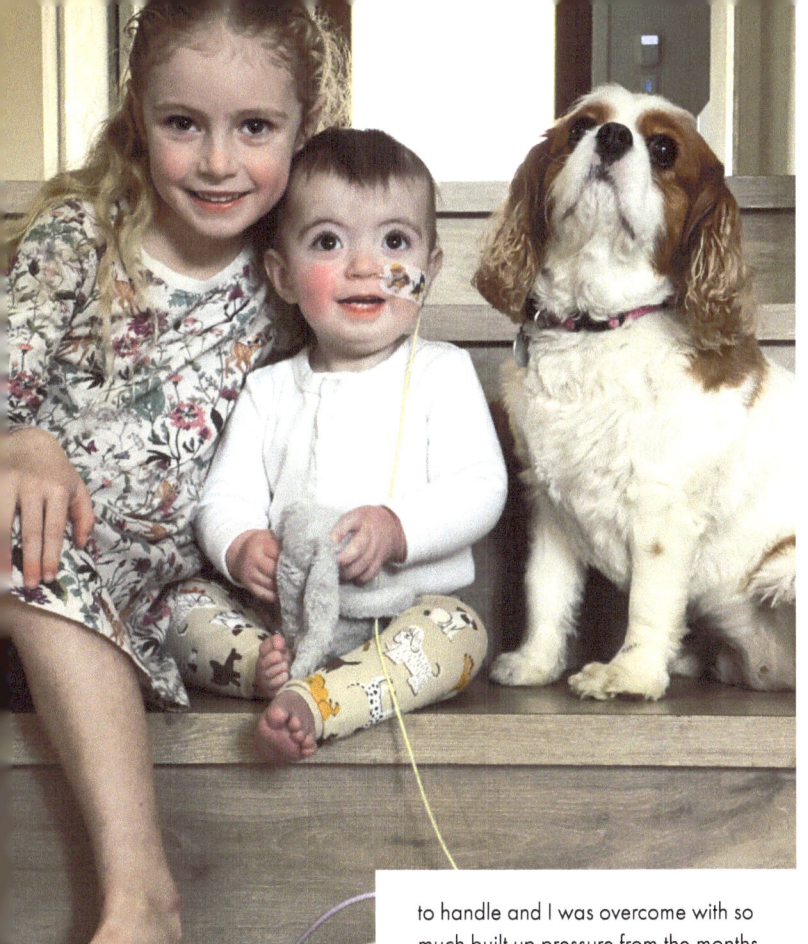

"It's all thanks to that tube that I got to bring Luke home and have him here today."

to handle and I was overcome with so much built up pressure from the months leading up to this day, the fear of how on Earth I was going to handle another big change and seeing Luke petrified. I was about to pass out and was quickly taken out of the operating room, leaving Luke still wide awake and scared. Hello mum guilt, you're back again!

I was comforted by a father of a 15-year-old girl. He brought me a tissue and told me he knew the feeling because he's an experienced medical parent and had been in my position many times before. We chatted while both our kids were in surgery. It was so humbling and reassuring to chat with a like-minded parent who just gets it.

Fast-forward to now, two weeks post-surgery, and Luke has completely come out of his shell. It's like he has a new lease on life! He has not stopped smiling and has quickly become quite an adventurous rascal. He's started putting food back into his mouth after weeks and weeks of refusing and his eyes have stopped continuously watering — something I questioned with many specialists who could never give me an answer. It breaks my heart to think that for the past 16 months he was uncomfortable.

The continual stares, feelings of being watched and invasion of personal space by curious children have also stopped. One of the best things? No more tube and tape changes! Besides the medical trauma, it's been a positive experience so far. Luke is happy and almost fully healed.

What advice do you have for parents who are new to tube-feeding? I had a lot of self-doubt about it, so to parents who are new to this, I'd say you're much more capable than you think. I'd also say to take each day as it comes and try to find acceptance. Tube-feeding is not the worst thing in the world. Without it I would have a very sick little boy — if I even had him at all. It's a bit brutal to think about it like that, but that's the reality of it. It's all thanks to that tube that I got to bring Luke home and have him here today.

---

thehandmadebabyboutique.com.au
@thehandmadebabyboutique
The Handmade Baby Boutique

the blend.

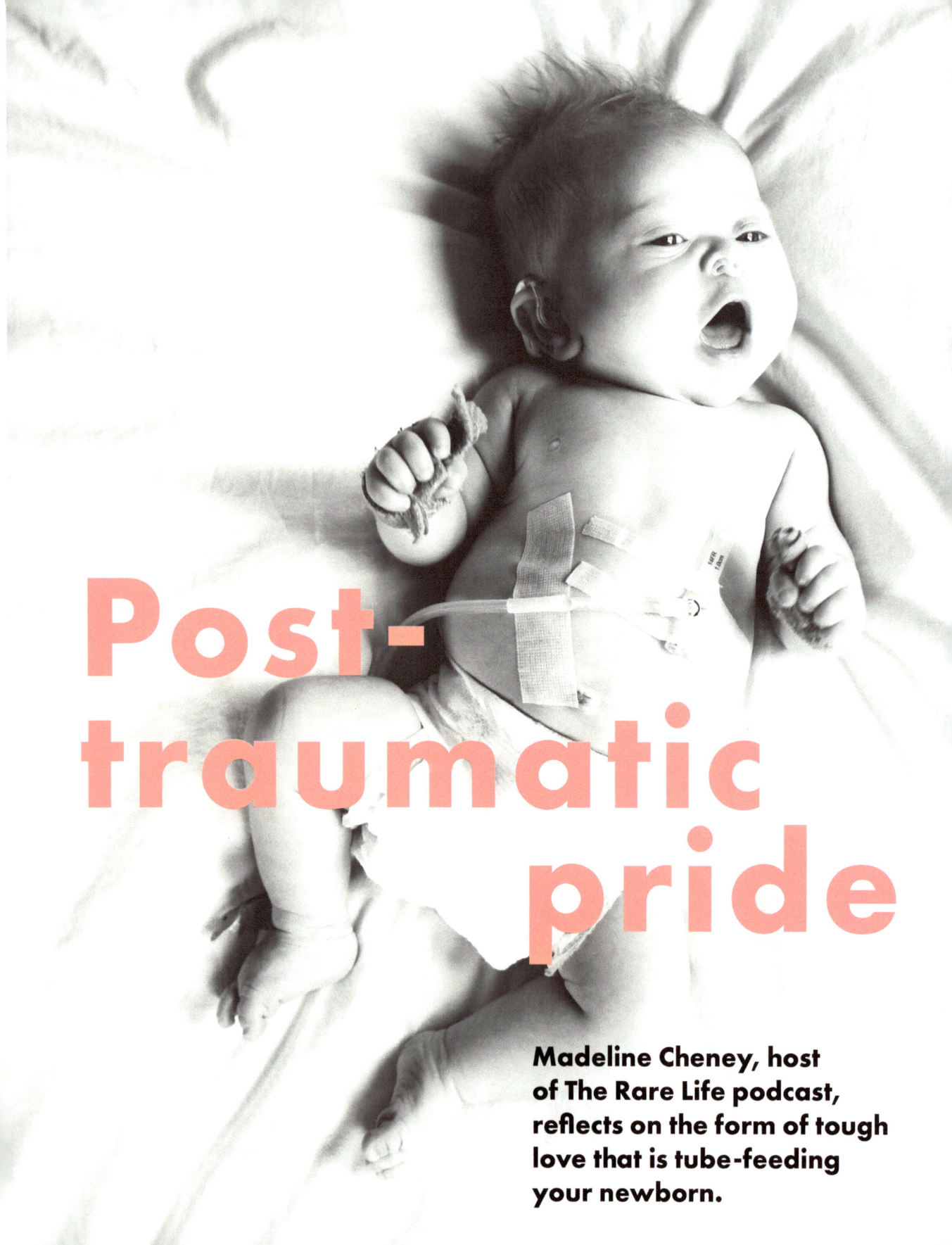

Post-traumatic pride

Madeline Cheney, host of The Rare Life podcast, reflects on the form of tough love that is tube-feeding your newborn.

/ **parent stories**

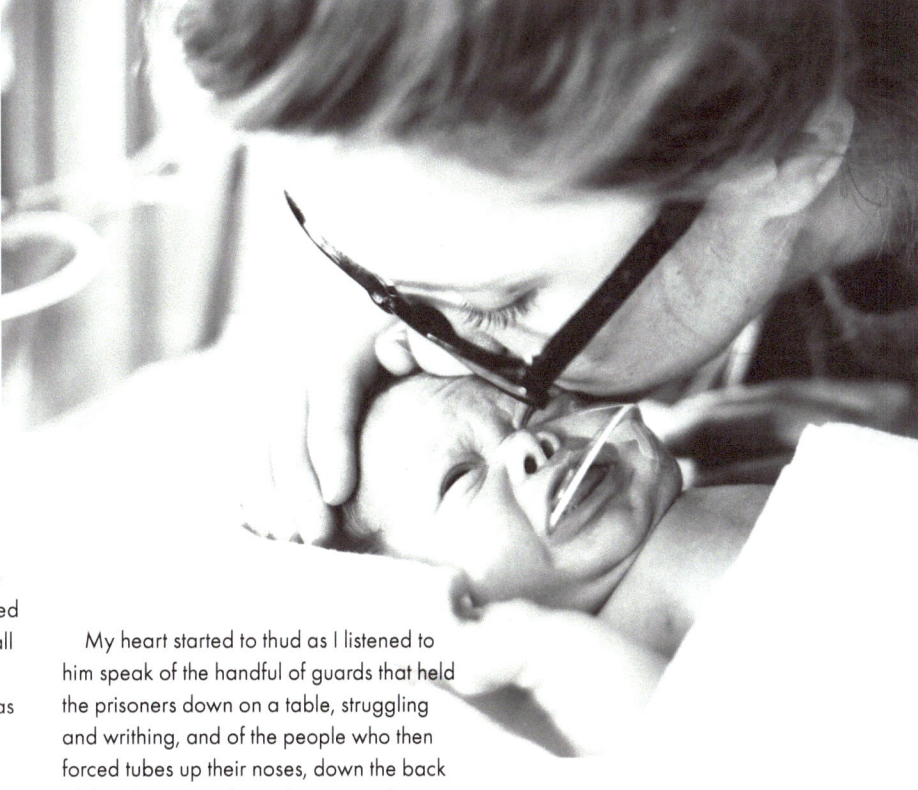

I was making the well-worn 30-minute drive home from the children's hospital we frequented for our infant son's care. Kimball was about six months old and buckled snug into his car seat as the radio played.

The station was National Public Radio (NPR) – as it always was in those early days.

Somehow it made me feel more connected to humanity to hear about politics and controversies. Using my brain in a way – any other way – than my constant striving to navigate the medical world and to understand a diagnosis so rare that Kimball's doctors had never heard of it.

I was vaguely aware that the radio host was telling a story about prisoners of war. My attention on the road and what had happened at that day's appointment brought his voice in and out of focus. Until he started to speak of hunger strikes and forced feeding via feeding tubes.

My heart started to thud as I listened to him speak of the handful of guards that held the prisoners down on a table, struggling and writhing, and of the people who then forced tubes up their noses, down the back of their throats, and into their stomachs.

He spoke of how incredibly painful this process is and likened it to torture.

My head reeled, my heart hammered harder and harder as what he was saying sunk in. The tears poured as I jabbed a shaking finger to the radio power button and left the car in a humming silence as I further processed it all.

My son.

My infant son.

Newborn and squirming and thrashing about as nurses held him down on his intensive care unit bed, another nurse threading a tiny tube into his mouth, down his throat, into his stomach.

The feeding pump sending pumped breast milk dripping into his round belly, me feeling grateful for a way to feed him. >>

the blend.

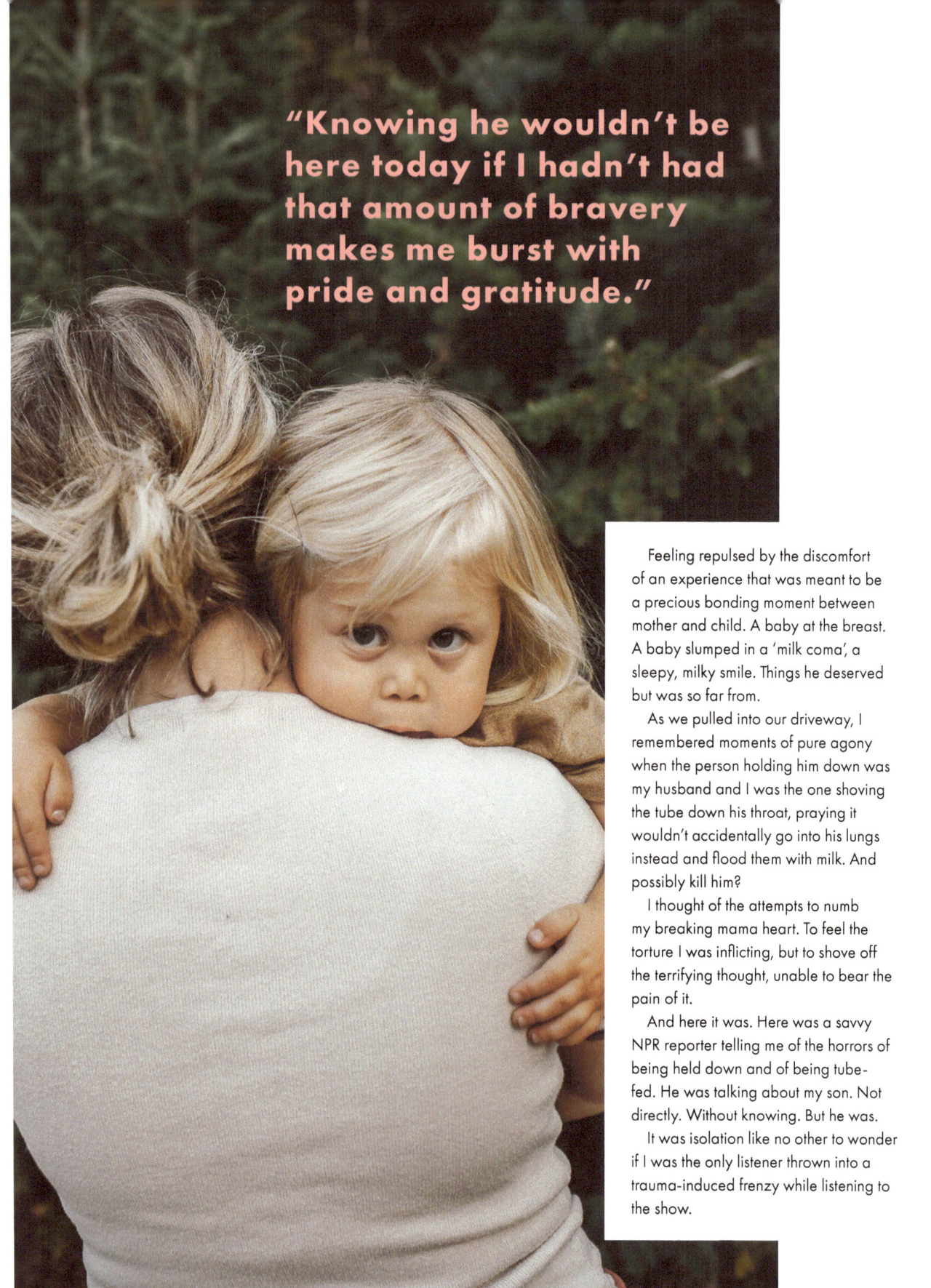

> "Knowing he wouldn't be here today if I hadn't had that amount of bravery makes me burst with pride and gratitude."

Feeling repulsed by the discomfort of an experience that was meant to be a precious bonding moment between mother and child. A baby at the breast. A baby slumped in a 'milk coma', a sleepy, milky smile. Things he deserved but was so far from.

As we pulled into our driveway, I remembered moments of pure agony when the person holding him down was my husband and I was the one shoving the tube down his throat, praying it wouldn't accidentally go into his lungs instead and flood them with milk. And possibly kill him?

I thought of the attempts to numb my breaking mama heart. To feel the torture I was inflicting, but to shove off the terrifying thought, unable to bear the pain of it.

And here it was. Here was a savvy NPR reporter telling me of the horrors of being held down and of being tube-fed. He was talking about my son. Not directly. Without knowing. But he was.

It was isolation like no other to wonder if I was the only listener thrown into a trauma-induced frenzy while listening to the show.

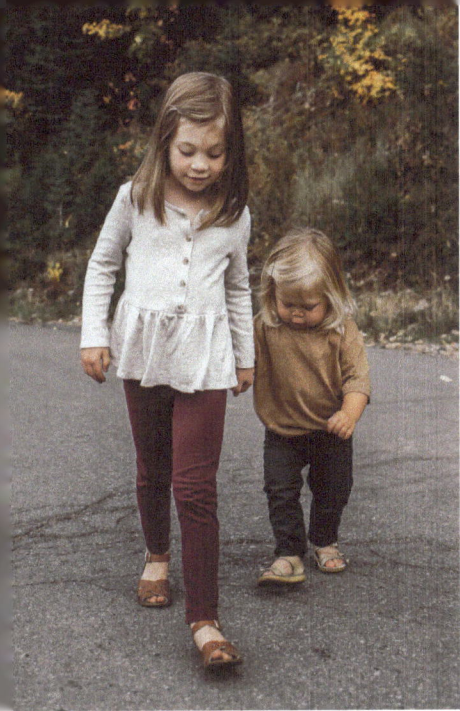

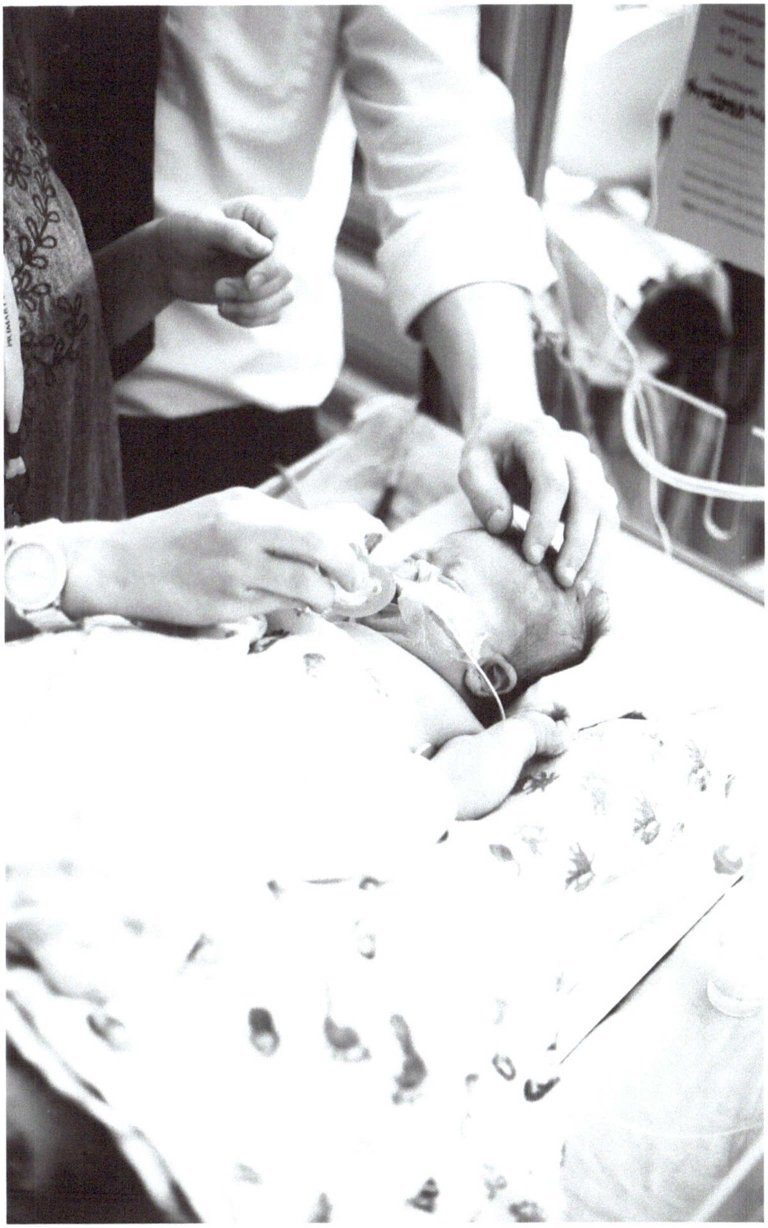

But now I know better. I know we are far from alone. I know there are other shaking fingers that would have jabbed at that radio button. I know there are countless other parents who are terrified about placing the tube incorrectly. Who are pumping their milk in an attempt to nurture their child in what seems to be the only way possible. Countless others rushing to the beeping pump, who have kitchen sinks full of syringes to be washed.

Kimball's four now. He's weaned from his tube and if he had it his way, he would still have the gastrostomy tube button he received surgically as a baby. Something he considered just as much a body part as his toes. He cried for weeks about its removal.

When I remember the days I had to torture my child in order to feed him, I still shudder. But knowing he wouldn't be here today if I hadn't had that amount of bravery makes me burst with pride and gratitude. Knowing I chose to do what brought us both terror so he could live a life full of giggles and Buzz Lightyear brings a depth to my motherhood I wouldn't have in any other way.

Madeline Cheney is the host and creator of The Rare Life, a much-loved podcast for parents of children with rare conditions. It can be binged on all podcasting platforms, Spotify, and at therarelifepodcast.com. Madeline is a fierce believer in the power of solidarity and of hot bubble baths with a good piece of historical fiction.

therarelifepodcast.com
@the_rare_life
The Rare Life Podcast

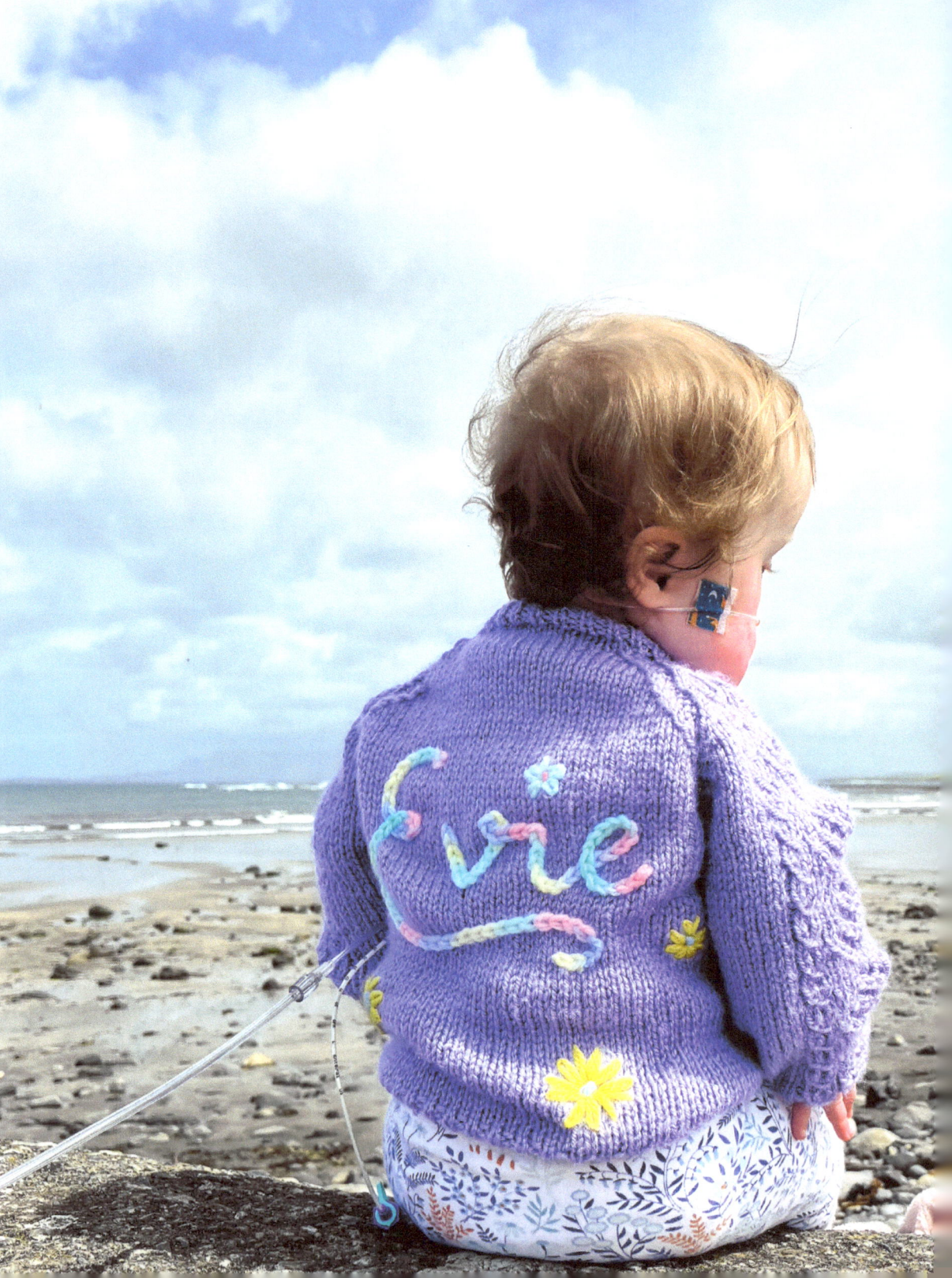

/ parent stories

A love like no other

A craic-loving couple are shouting their daughter's worth and showing the world how much fun can be had by a tube-feeding family. Introducing Brana Gadsby, Ross Worth and their beautiful Evie.

Brana and Ross were not expecting to be able to celebrate their daughter Evie's first birthday. During Brana's pregnancy, a scan revealed their baby had serious heart issues, leaving the first-time parents with a dire prognosis. Speaking from their home on the west coast of Ireland, just days before Evie turns one, the pair admit they are 'very emotional'.

'It's amazing to see her so well on her first birthday,' Brana says, nestled with Ross while bouncing a distractingly cute Evie on her lap. 'It's better than we could have ever imagined.'

Brana is a nurse and had guessed that Evie, who has Down syndrome, might have trouble feeding. She and Ross were warned their baby would likely experience heart failure at six weeks old – which she did. An NG (nasogastric) tube was placed soon after. >>

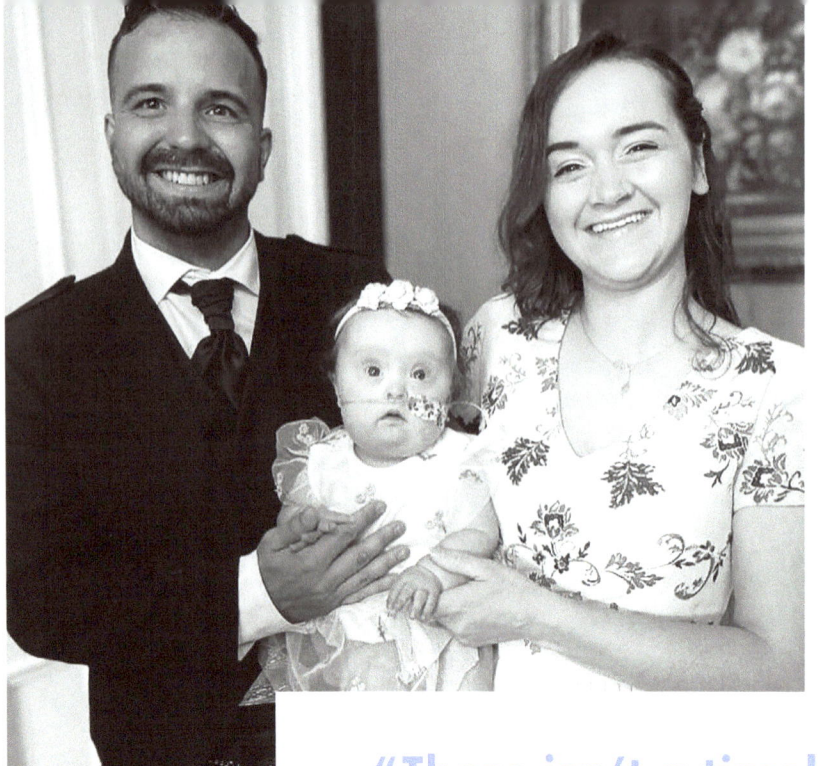

'There was a lot of relief for us when the tube went in. We were in a constant cycle of trying to get her to feed or trying to get her to sleep,' says Ross, turning to Evie. 'Which was sad, because you wanted to do things other than just sleeping and feeding. When the tube went in it was much easier for us and she could actually just enjoy being a baby.'

'And that was the main thing for us,' says Brana. 'We didn't know how long we would have with her. So enjoying that time with her and interacting with her was so important.'

Evie's first year has been full of adventures. Beachcombing and mountain-climbing near home, and road-tripping to Scotland in the Volkswagen Crafter her parents converted into a cosy campervan.

Her first sojourn in this van saw Brana and Ross accidentally melting her milk bottles ('we thought sterilisation required steaming') but the pair have since mastered tube-feeding on the go – opting for gravity feeds over a pump ('a pump is just extra gear') and keeping elastic bands handy for hanging syringes.

Evie now eats a range of meals orally – despite a false start on the solid food.

'I was really excited when she turned six months old because I was like, great, now we can begin solids,' says Brana. 'That lasted about two weeks before she started getting stressed out. Then I got really stressed out. It just wasn't working.'

Evie's development is behind that of her typically-developing peers.

'So for her to start weaning at six months was probably too soon – even though she was interested in the food that we were eating,' says Brana.

Evie took a break from the solids and tried again a few months later.

'I was like, you lead us, because it stressed me out so much and I was getting really, really bummed out about it,' says Brana. 'Now her eating is going really well and I think it's because we followed her lead. There isn't a timeline for people who don't fit the "normal" criteria, so you need to be really clued into your child and not pressured from the outside.'

Nowadays Evie enjoys a mix of solids supplemented by formula tube-feeds. Her NG tube has, for the most part, stayed in place.

'I rolled over in bed and whipped it out once by accident!' says Brana. 'But Evie really isn't grabby. I've also learnt to tape very close to the nostril because she would get her little finger in and flick it out.'

Brana's the expert on taping, as was made clear when she got Covid and Ross – a software engineer – stepped in and fashioned a web of tape across Evie's face. The family shares such shenanigans on their YouTube vlog and Instagram account. >>

> "There isn't a timeline for people who don't fit the 'normal' criteria, so you need to be really clued into your child and not pressured from the outside."

/ parent stories

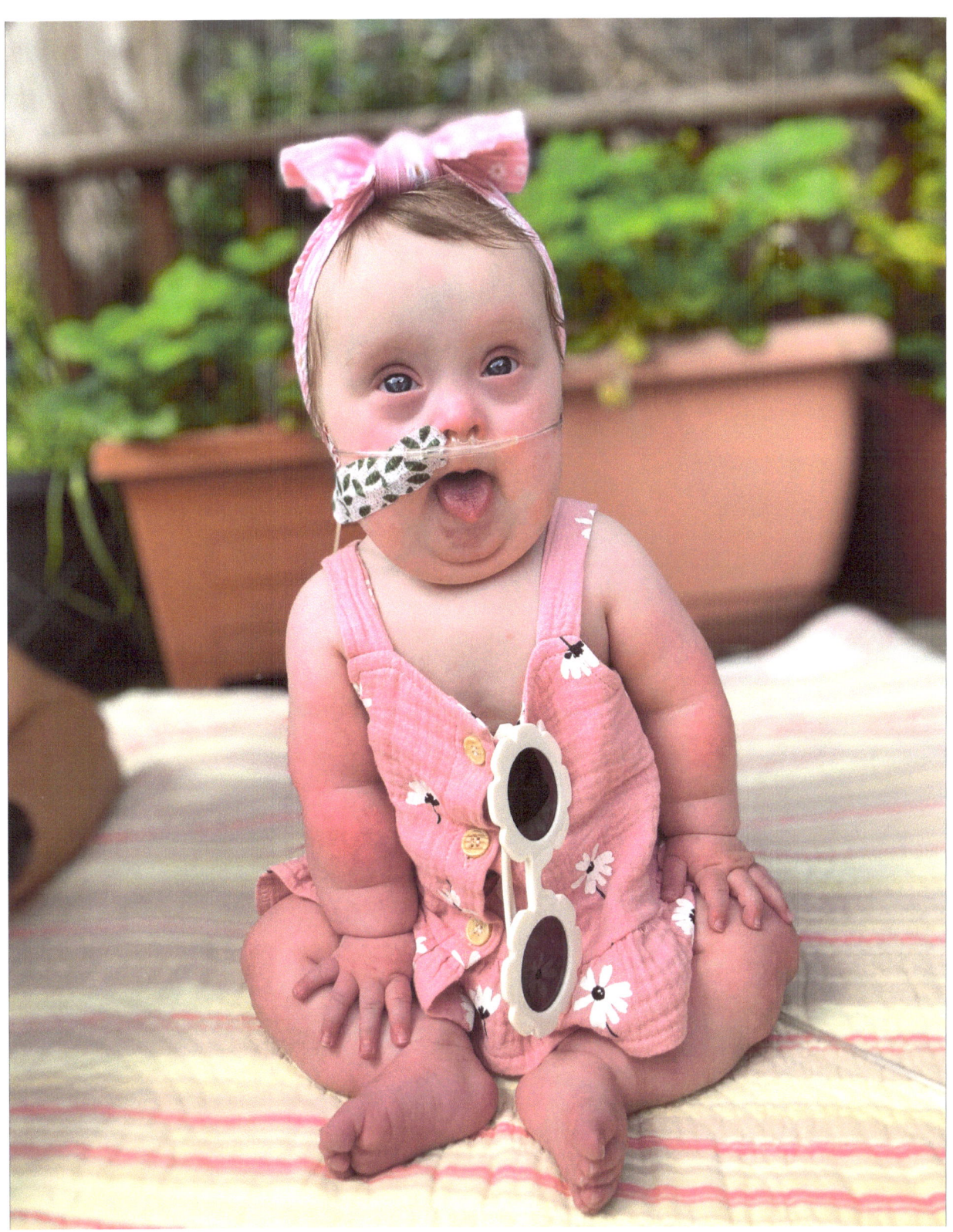

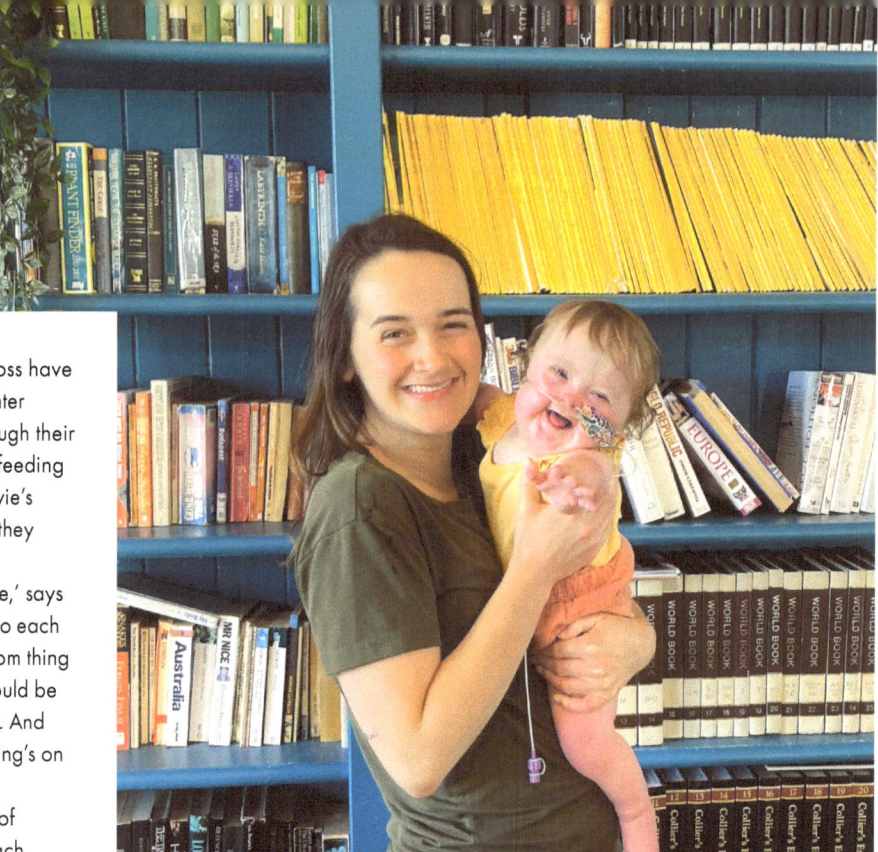

While the love Brana and Ross have for each other and their daughter radiates, heartwarmingly, through their videos and posts, fellow tube-feeding parents might wonder, amid Evie's many medical needs, how do they sustain their relationship?

'We communicate all the time,' says Brana. 'We never stop talking to each other. It could be about a random thing that pops into our head, or it could be something more deep than that. And timing doesn't matter. If something's on our mind, we'll just shout it out.'

'We're also very conscious of showing how much we love each other,' says Ross. 'Sometimes things do get stressful or hard and if we get snappy, we're quick to recognise it in ourselves and apologise for it. Even before Evie was here, when we first got together we recognised how much of a good team we make. We're always on each other's side.'

Like many of us whose children are not following typical paths, Brana and Ross often find people telling them things like, 'I couldn't do what you do'.

'But you could,' says Ross, offering some words of advice to parents who are new to tube-feeding. 'You're going to love this child more than anything and you are going to do whatever you can so that they're comfortable and they're happy.'

'We didn't wake up here with tubes and wires and machines and equipment and appointments – we were led into this,' adds Brana. 'We didn't choose to be in this position, but we're over the moon that we are here.'

By the time this story goes to print, Evie will have welcomed a sister who may well not need to tube-feed.

'I'm so excited about breastfeeding, because I really enjoyed that while it lasted with Evie,' says Brana. 'I'm trying not to big it up too much just in case it doesn't happen – breastfeeding is not always an easy journey, I know that – but I love the idea of just whipping your boob out and feeding your baby.'

Ross is also looking forward to the convenience of potentially straight-forward bottle-feeding, but thinks having a baby who isn't Evie 'will just be weird'.

'I am excited for it, but when I'm holding other babies they're so wriggly and constantly doing things, whereas Evie's so gentle and chilled out. She's so lovely and I just love her so much.'

Followers of the family will know that Ross and Brana own three almost identical dogs – all border-collie crosses. 'They look the same, they act mostly the same, and I just want that with my kids too,' laughs Ross, smiling at Evie. 'I want them all to be the same, you're great.'

---

shoutingeviesworth.com
@shouting_eviesworth
Ross+Brana

'Our kids come as they are. Now it's up to us to get with the program.'

Melanie Dimmitt, *Special: Antidotes to the obsessions that come with a child's disability.*

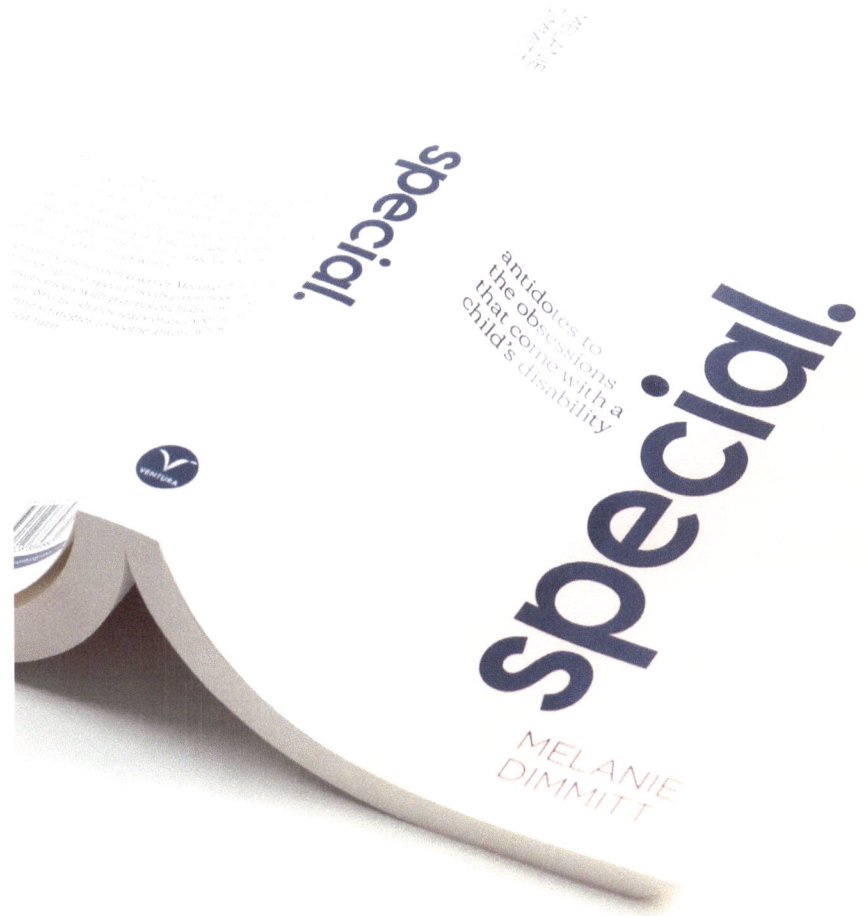

Available to purchase online at all good booksellers.

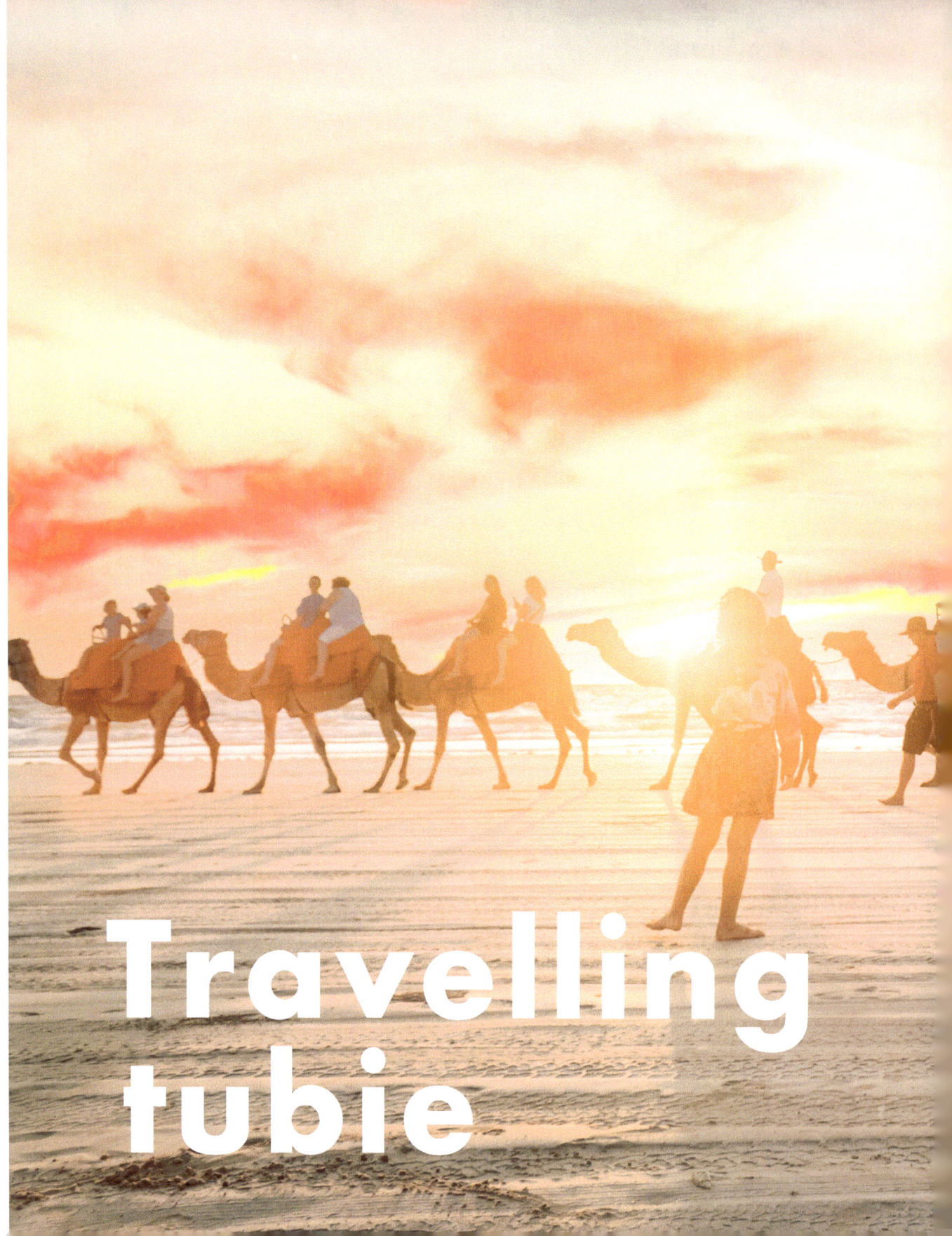

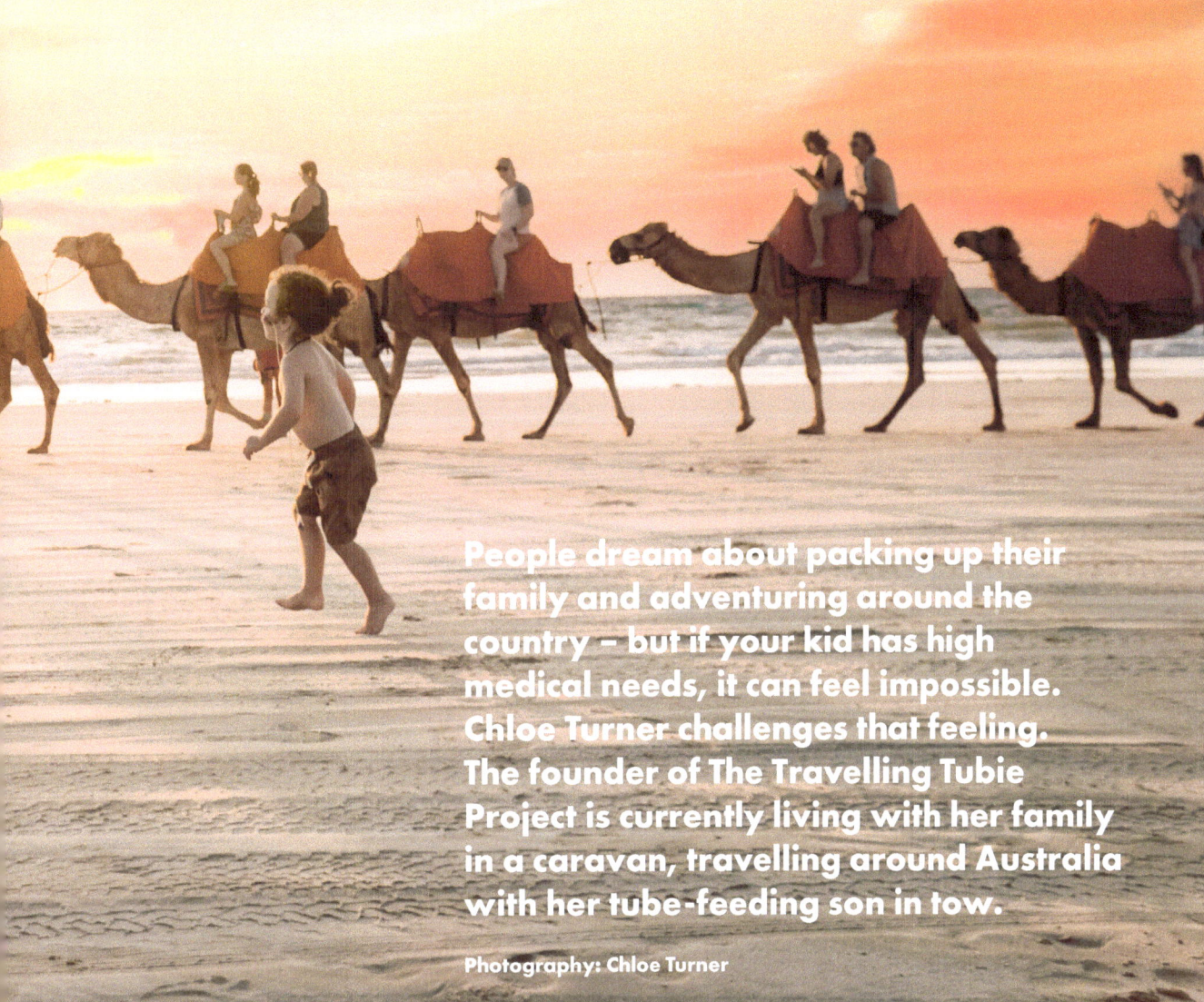

People dream about packing up their family and adventuring around the country – but if your kid has high medical needs, it can feel impossible. Chloe Turner challenges that feeling. The founder of The Travelling Tubie Project is currently living with her family in a caravan, travelling around Australia with her tube-feeding son in tow.

Photography: Chloe Turner

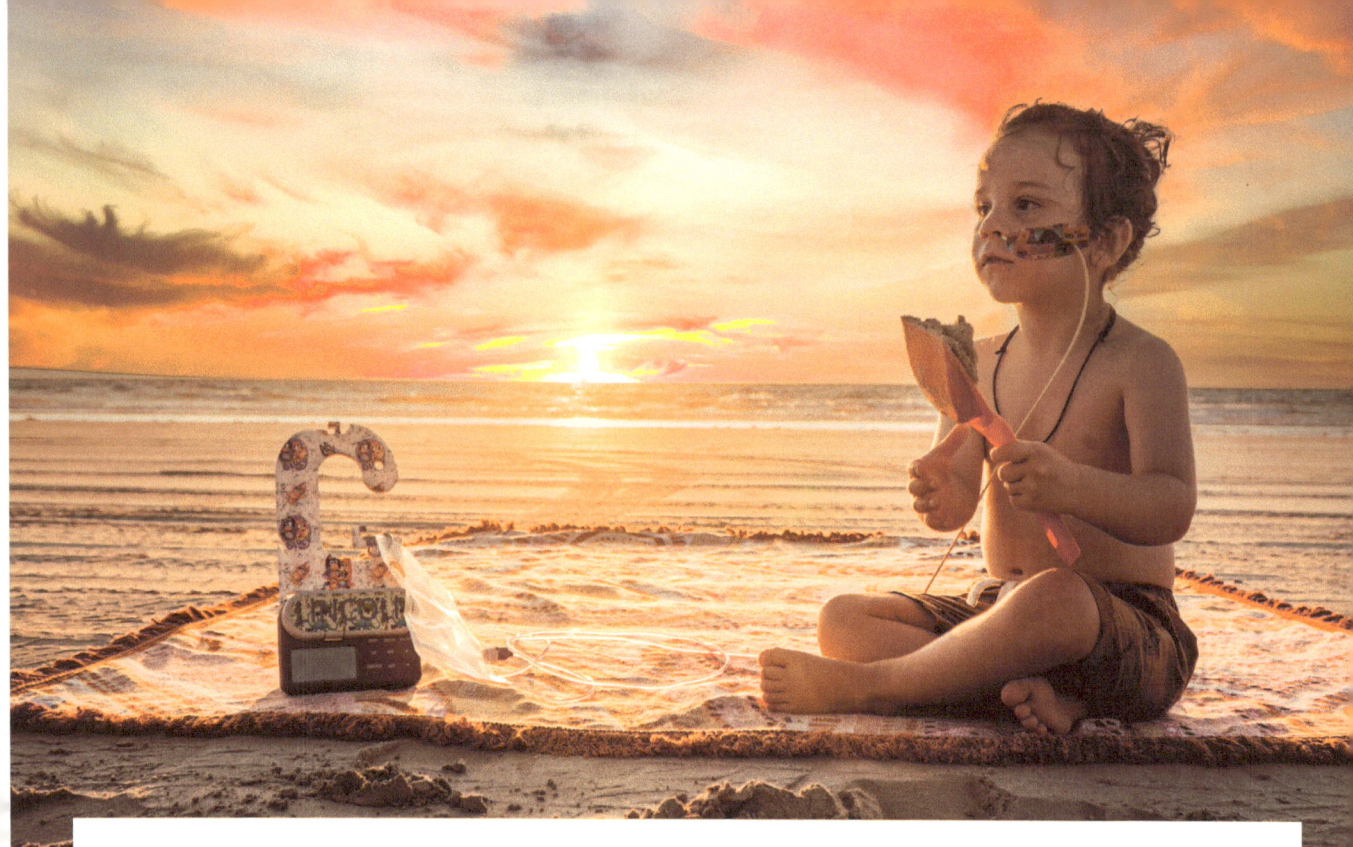

So many people questioned us about uprooting our family. Paediatricians gave my son Lincoln the all-clear, medically speaking, while warning us that he wouldn't have opportunities to socialise. But he's gone from being a shy little toddler who would hide behind my legs to a kid that says, 'Mum, there's a new friend!' He'll suss out other caravans and say, 'Mum, bikes! Mum, friends!'

Before we hit the road, my husband, Shaun, and I weren't in a good place. We'd been through a lot with Lincoln who has several medical issues but, as yet, no diagnosis. We were also in a load of debt from his medical bills and, with life constantly being disrupted, we were struggling to hold down jobs.

It got to the point where Shaun and I just looked at each other and said, 'what are we doing?'. We felt like we were just trying to survive. We weren't getting anywhere. We weren't achieving anything. What we really – and always had – wanted to do, was travel.

Then I went away with the kids for a week while Shaun worked. I just needed to get out of the house – it was raining, it was winter, it was awful. So we went away and something incredible happened. Lincoln slept. This is a kid who we usually have to medicate to sleep, but he went to sleep with the sun and woke up with the sun. He let me get him dressed, he let me change his nappy and he was happy. He was a different kid. And I thought, we just need to do this.

Lincoln was well at the time – he'd weaned off his nasogastric (NG) tube.

> "So we went away and something incredible happened. Lincoln slept. This is a kid who we usually have to medicate to sleep, but he went to sleep with the sun and woke up with the sun."

But the real clincher was when Shaun walked in our front door one day and said, 'the carport is bloody flooded again, let's do it'.

So we started telling people. We told my parents over drinks at our local

/ feature

pub and Mum said, 'gosh, I have a friend who did that. I haven't seen her in a couple of years but I'll shoot her a message'. I kid you not, that woman walked in the pub door five minutes later. We spent the next hour quizzing her about how she did it with young kids. Hearing how much her children thrived while travelling, we knew we had to do it.

Meanwhile, our good friend's brother heard we wanted to sell our house. He did a walkthrough of our place and, two weeks later, it was sold. We got rid of all of our stuff, paid off our debts and bought a caravan. We were homeless, but happy. Once we set off – westward from Adelaide – our stress disappeared.

Our caravan is on the luxury end as we wanted to be comfortable. You can't be in the middle of nowhere without a toilet, especially with kids toilet training! Having our own bathroom means we can go off-grid, as we do often. A recent highlight was spending a week in Western Australia's Karijini National Park.

The park is about three-and-a-half hours from Port Hedland and it's full of gorges that have been carved out of the land by spring-fed water. There are waterfalls and swimming holes filled with fish. Both kids faced their fears of tiny fish nibbling at their feet and went swimming. There are dingoes around, too. I saw my first wild dingo, which was on my bucket list. Next to tick off is swimming with crocs in Lake Argyle.

We took the child-hiking carrier to Karijini because Lincoln doesn't have a great amount of stamina, but he's a natural climber. We were doing class-five hikes – which is the highest level you can do without a guide – and Lincoln was scrambling down gorges like they were ladders.

When we came back to Port Hedland, one of our caravan park neighbours told me, 'you're glowing'. I felt so replenished. We're now settled for four weeks of fishing, swimming every day and working before heading off again for three months to Darwin.

I help Lincoln's sister, Grace, with her distance education during the day so I'm working night-fill at Woolworths. They're happy to have me for whatever hours I want to work and it's not an issue if I need to duck off midway through a shift when Lincoln is sick. Now that I'm on their payroll, I can walk into any Woolies around the country and start work within a week. >>

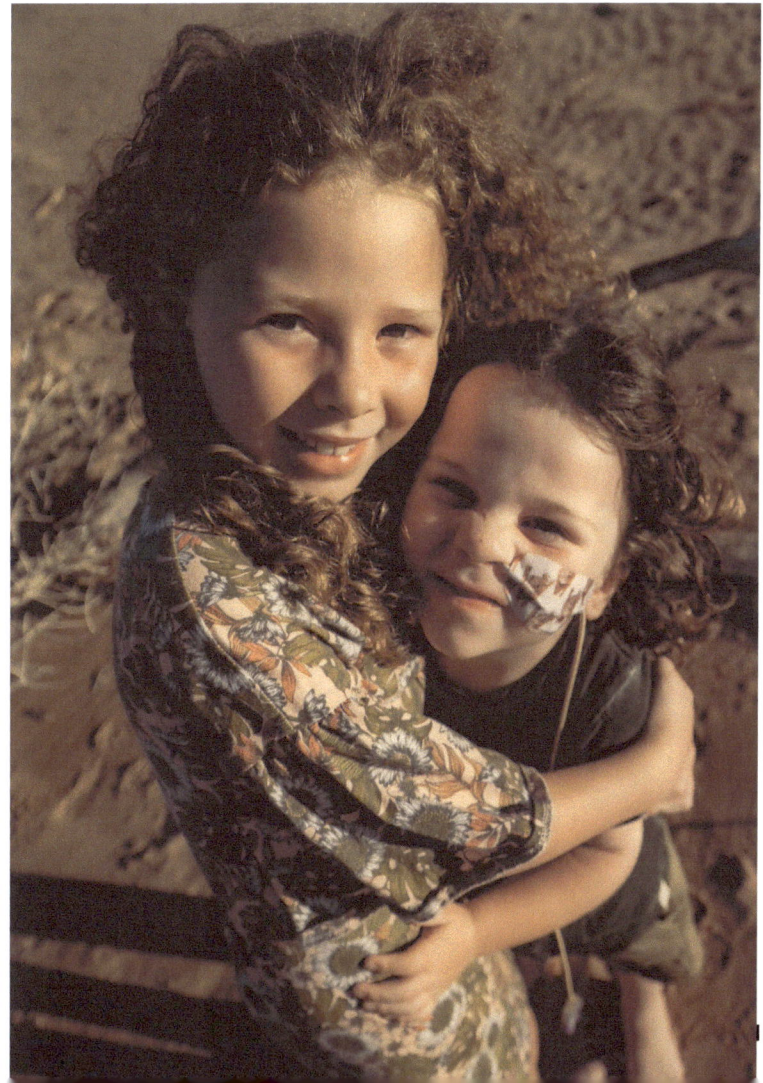

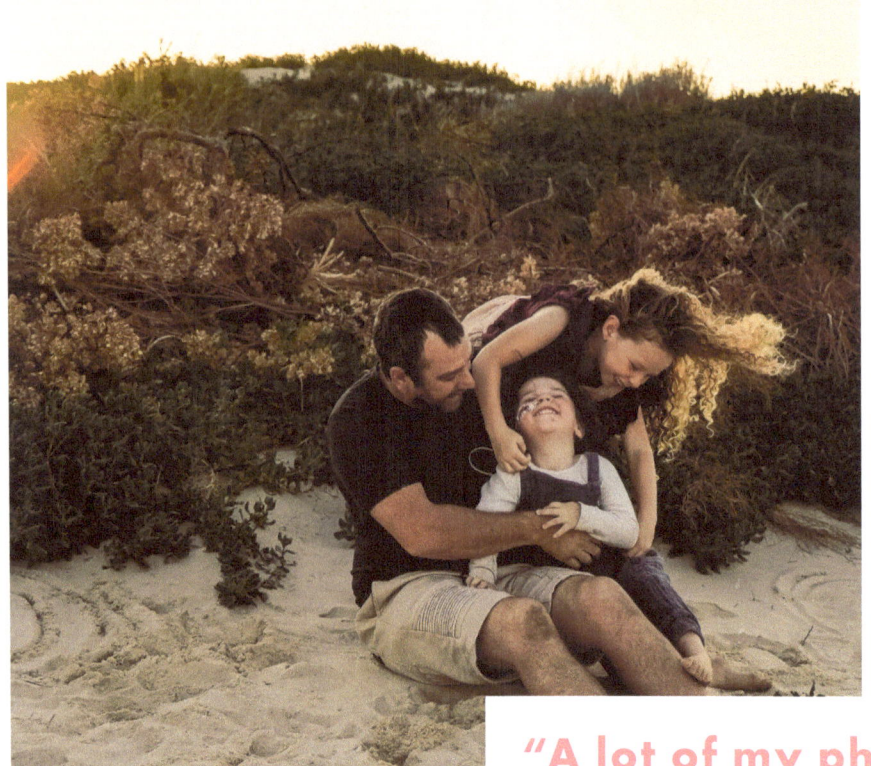

I jumped on the Mighty Mums' Perth Facebook group and said: 'Can anyone help me? I can return the favour by taking photos of your family for free!'

The families I photographed in Perth all have vastly different stories. The first family I met with belonged to Amiyah, a terminally ill child. This family was so welcoming and so loving towards their daughter. I'd walked in so nervous – and left with my heart full.

> "A lot of my photos have a sun flare or a little rainbow in them. I feel like that says, here's your little bit of hope. You've made it through this."

I've also got my online tube-feeding accessories store, The Travelling Tubie Project, ticking away thanks to a fellow medical mum I hired to take care of the operations back home in Adelaide. We recently had a three-hour Zoom meeting about our new pump hangers which I'm so excited for. It's a great partnership and she does an incredible job.

Being on the road has allowed me to get creative and build out a new arm of the business. I'd always wanted to do photography and one night before we set off it hit me – I could meet and photograph tubie families as we travel around.

With no diagnosis, I've always felt that Lincoln – and our family – doesn't have a space to belong. Well, why can't we just make that space? If you've got or have had a tube, it doesn't matter why you've got it, you can be a part of this. That was the plan behind my project and it's led me to so many lovely families.

Our travels have had to be slow. We were supposed to have lapped the whole country by now but we've only done Western Australia. That's actually been a blessing because we've been able to dive deeper into communities and get to know people better.

Lincoln has had some health troubles so his NG has made a return. Had this happened at home, I would've sunk back into a bad place. On the road, it just felt like a speed bump.

Thankfully I met some mums in Perth who sorted us out, because we didn't have any tube-feeding supplies.

Another family booked a studio for our shoot – which was a first for me – and we managed to tear the backdrop. We got some great captures regardless and I ushered the family outside for some golden-hour shots. That's really become my thing. A lot of my photos have a sun flare or a little rainbow in them. I feel like that says, here's your little bit of hope, you've made it through this.

The family that booked the studio has a little girl on total parenteral nutrition (TPN) and she's got a G-tube as well. She was lots of fun – so giggly and funny. I got some beautiful photos of her holding her pump pole and the sun was just peeking through from behind her head. >>

/ feature

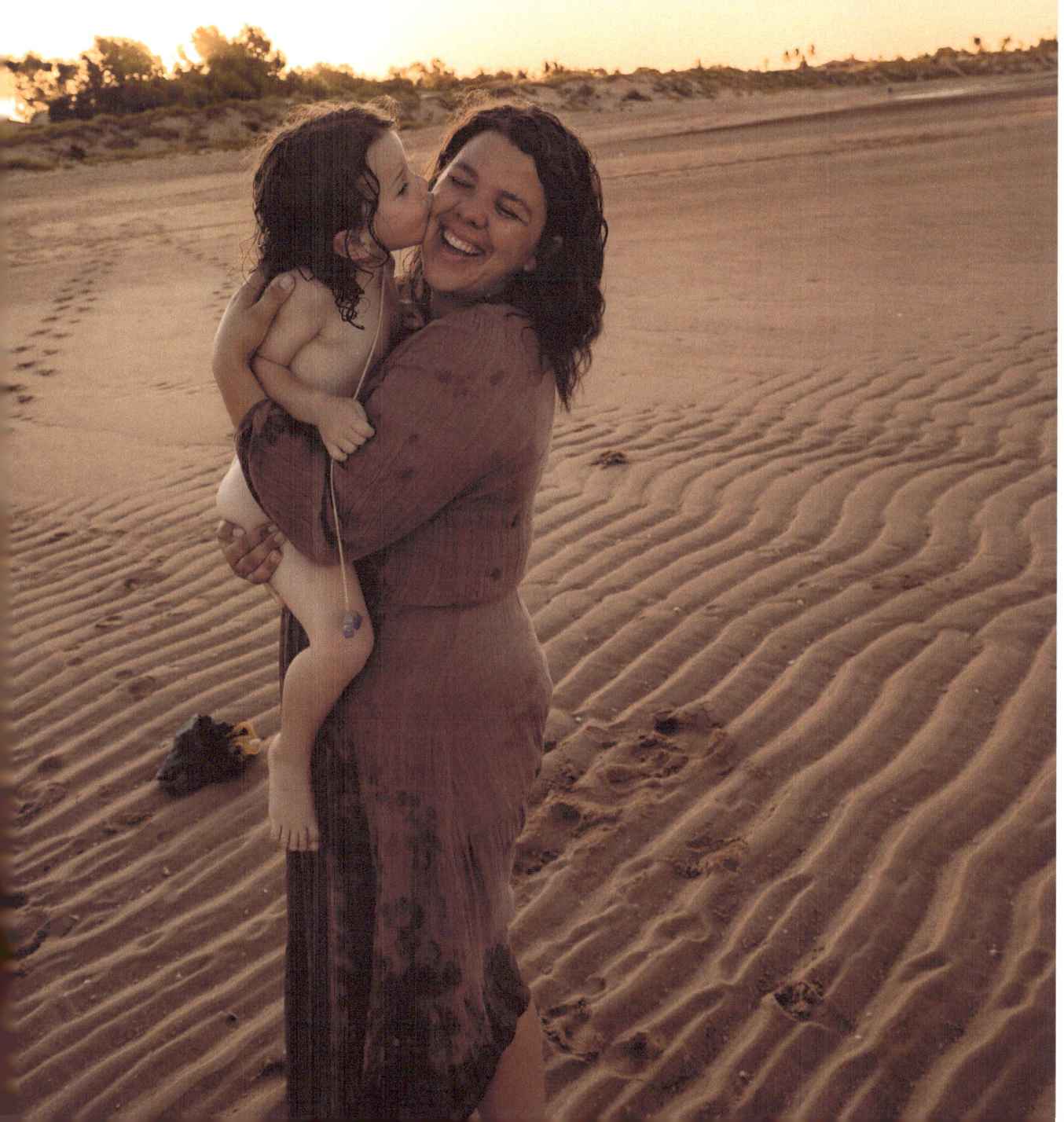

There was another little girl in a wheelchair and she was a bit trickier to photograph. But once Mum got her giggling and moving around, her face just lit up. Everyone I've met has been so happy, so joyful.

A few families have told me they've tried to work with other photographers – ones who don't have any knowledge of tube-feeding or disabilities – and it's been awful, uncomfortable and at times even unsafe. That's really spurred me on to keep doing this.

We've been on the road a year now and will keep travelling – on to Broome, Kununurra and Darwin next – as long as Lincoln's health lets us. We're having so much fun and even when things have gotten hairy, we've managed. Most of the time, the curve-balls have given us great stories to tell.

While we were snorkelling in Exmouth, Lincoln got an ear infection, so we got him on antibiotics. Once he seemed better, we felt reassured enough to head to our next destination, Giralia Station, an outback setting along the Coral Coast that, as we would discover, is only accessible via almost 30km of corrugated road.

It was beautiful there – riddled with turtles – but by our second night, Lincoln wasn't looking great. His temperature started to spike at 40C and we couldn't get it down with Panadol and Nurofen. So we woke early one morning, packed everything up, drove the bloody 30 corrugated kilometres at 10km/h to get out and continued for seven hours straight to the hospital in Karratha. The last two hours were the toughest, by far.

Once admitted we found out he had two antibiotic-resistant viruses, so I'm glad we made that choice. There have been a few times we've had to pack up and hightail it to a hospital because Lincoln has needed something. We've got vital signs monitors in the caravan, so we can monitor him, but there are times when our guts tell us we've gotta get going.

Lincoln's tube has been in and out. It's in again now and when I got back to the caravan after Lincoln had it re-inserted, I was pretty devastated. I said to Shaun,

> "We're having so much fun and even when things have gotten hairy, we've managed. Most of the time, the curve-balls have given us great stories to tell."

'I feel like I have to torture our child to make him feel better'.

But then I heard Shaun speaking to our neighbours about Lincoln's tube. 'He's had it before,' Shaun said. 'He knows what to do.' The neighbours asked, 'can he still play?' And Shaun said, 'can he ever'. This kid hangs from trees a lot of the time, so we just have to make sure he tucks it in so he doesn't pull it out – which he's done before! He can still go swimming. He can still do everything. If anything, the tube makes this possible.

Listening to Shaun gave me the pep talk I needed. I'd only just gotten used to people not staring again and I thought Lincoln's friends were going to freak out. But they just said 'oh cool' and kept playing.

We've learnt a lot on this trip and it's reconnected us as a family. We've grown closer and have started to heal from the trauma we went through with Lincoln. I hope we can inspire other families raising kids with medical needs to travel and do things that they might think are impossible.

For those who want to travel, I'd advise planning ahead, knowing which hospitals have 24-hour emergency departments along the way and having spare gear and meds on board just in case. You don't always have to go far. The very first trip we took was only 45 minutes from our local children's hospital – and it was one of our favourites. There are ways to escape the daily grind while keeping our kids safe.

This opportunity has given us so much and I've met such inspiring families, all while doing things I'm passionate about. I never felt I had a place, until now.

---

tubieproject.com
@the.travelling.tubie.project
The Travelling Tubie Project

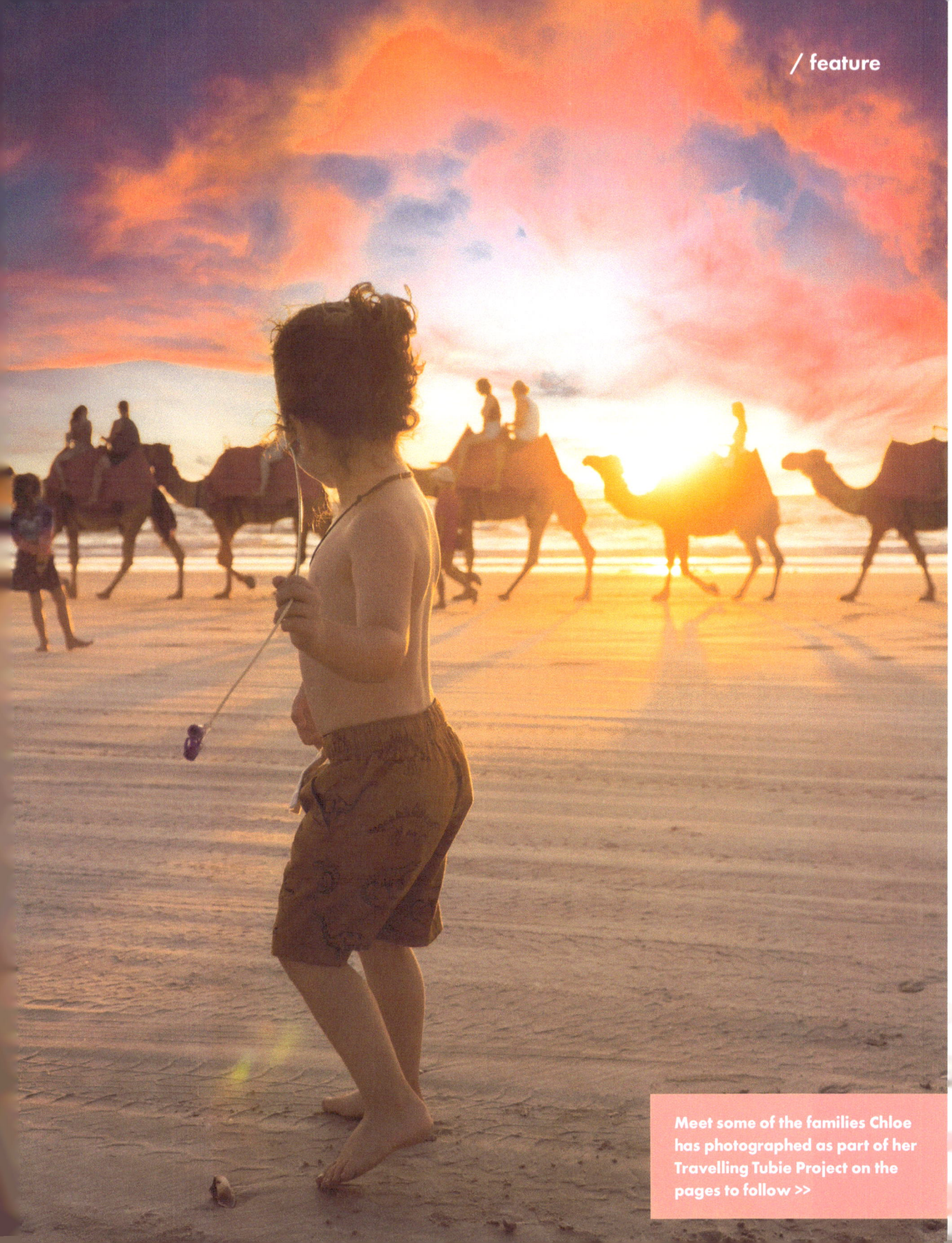

/ feature

Meet some of the families Chloe has photographed as part of her Travelling Tubie Project on the pages to follow >>

Everleigh's mum, Stacy

'Tube-feeding is daunting and unfamiliar initially – which can be frightening and intimidating. But you'll adapt quickly. You'll learn a new set of skills and a new vocabulary you didn't even know existed. And you'll find a new norm for your family. Find your new community that is going to listen, understand and be your rock throughout your journey.'

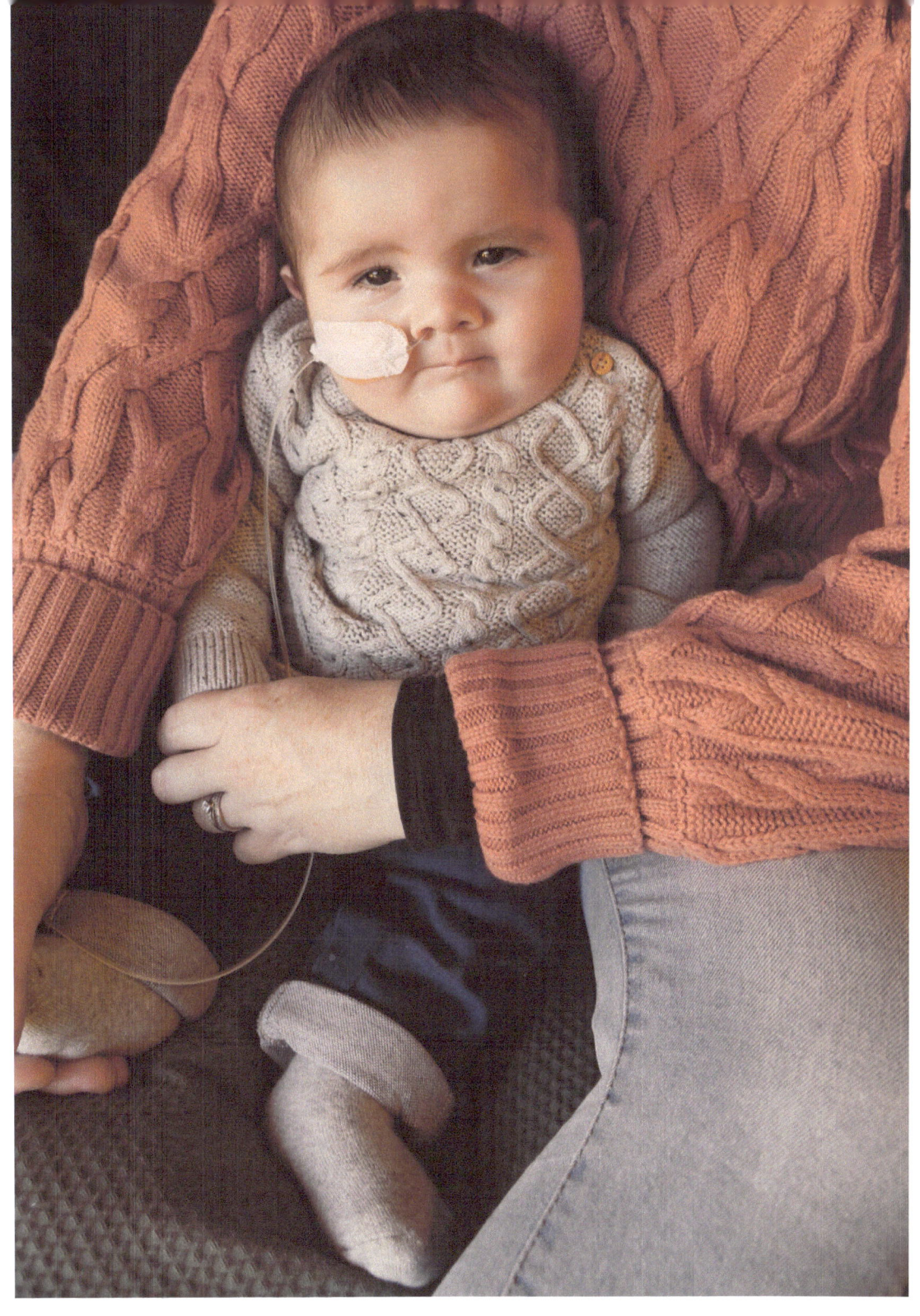

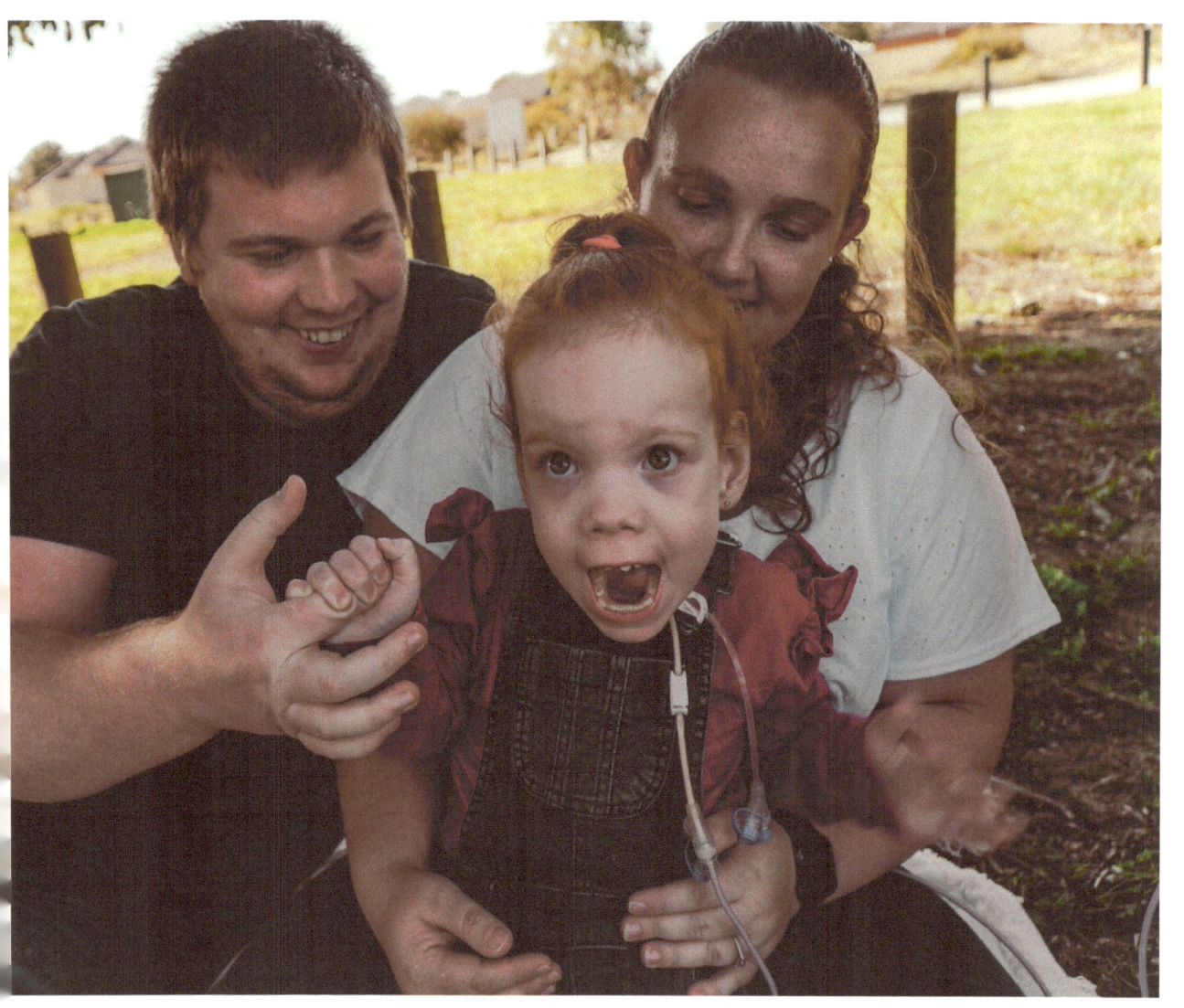

Gabriella's mum, Toni

'It's scary to start tube-feeding your child, but don't panic. You're not alone in your tube-feeding journey. Try and stay focused on the positives. Fed is best, no matter how you get your food.'

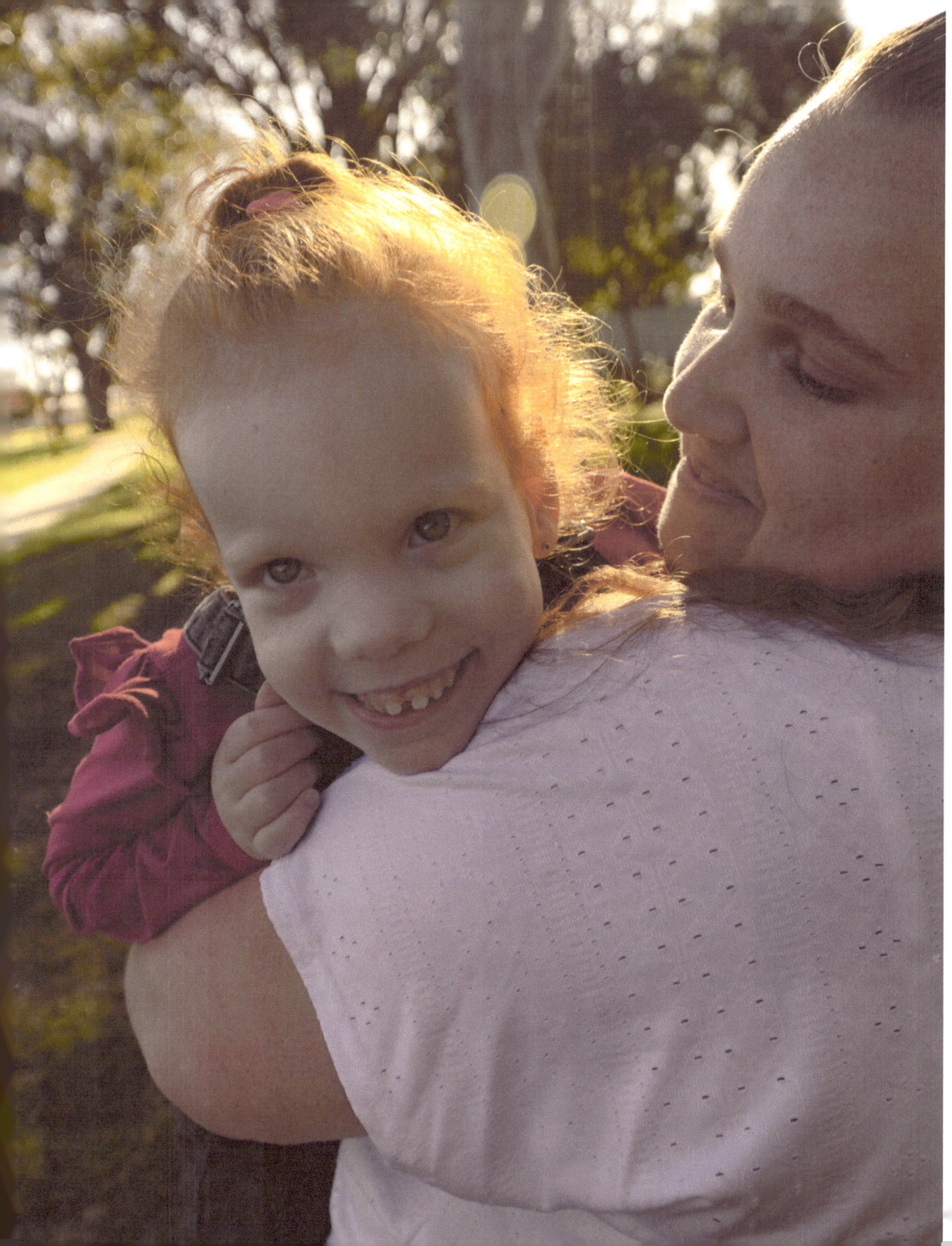

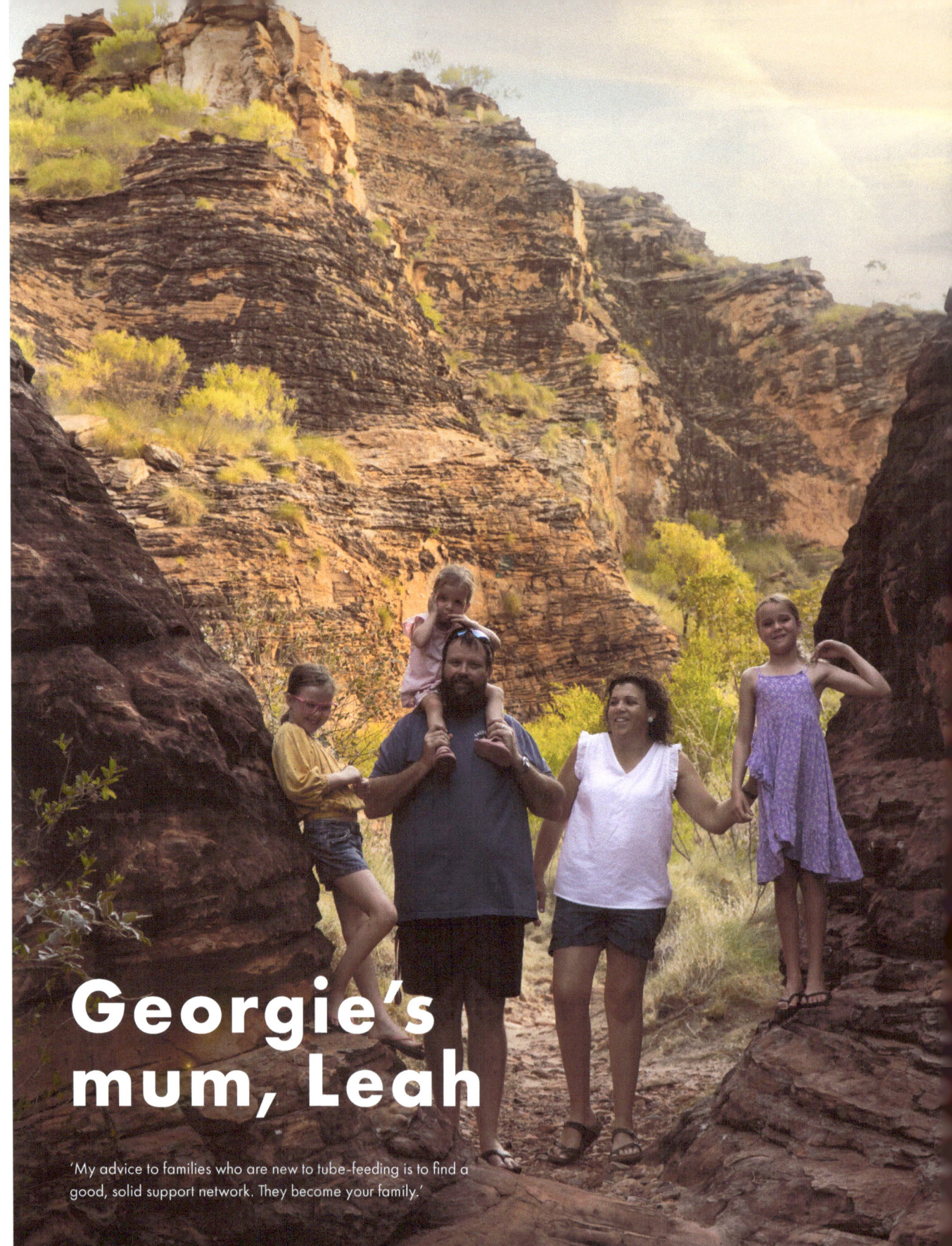

Georgie's mum, Leah

'My advice to families who are new to tube-feeding is to find a good, solid support network. They become your family.'

/ photo series

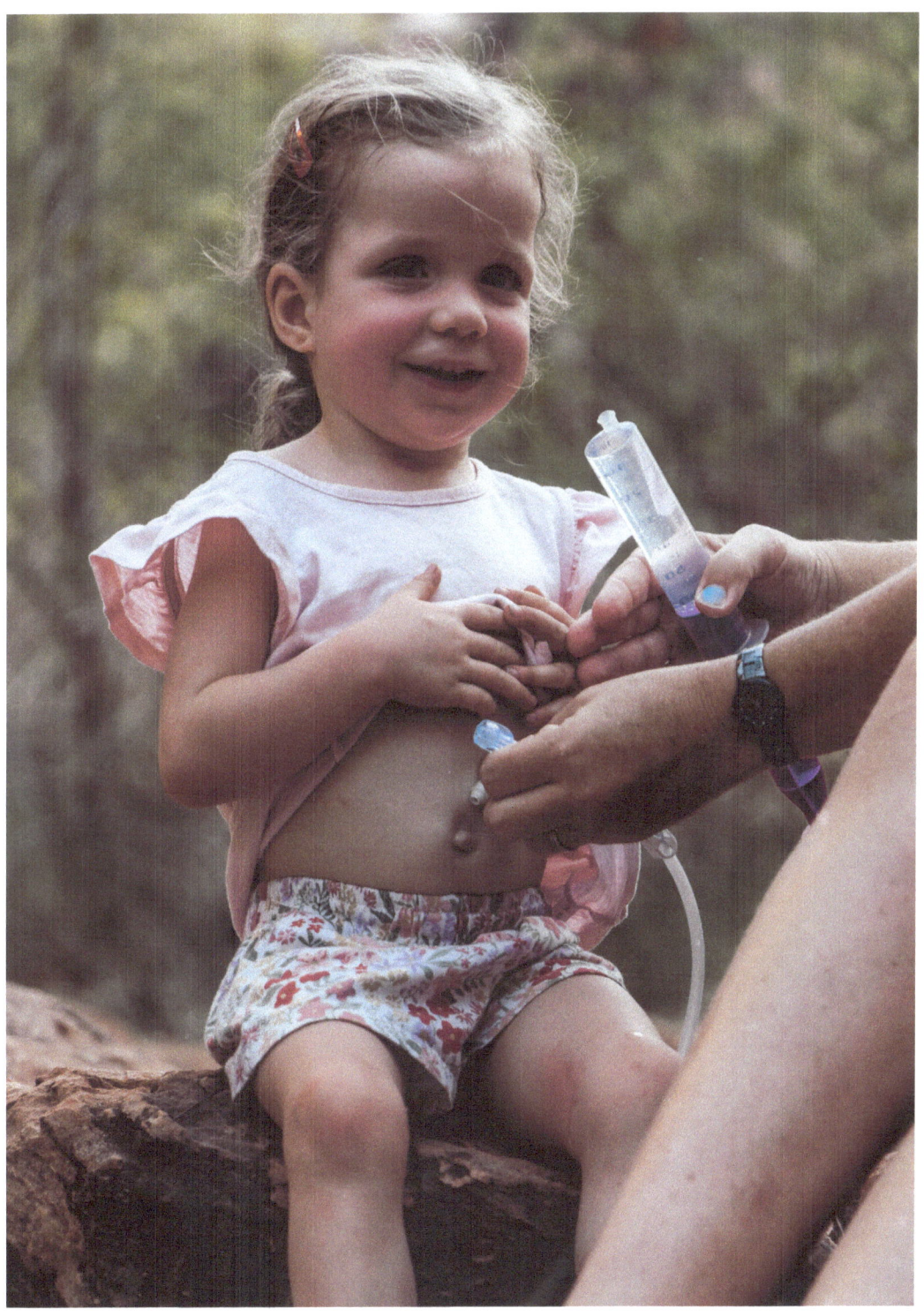

the blend.   111

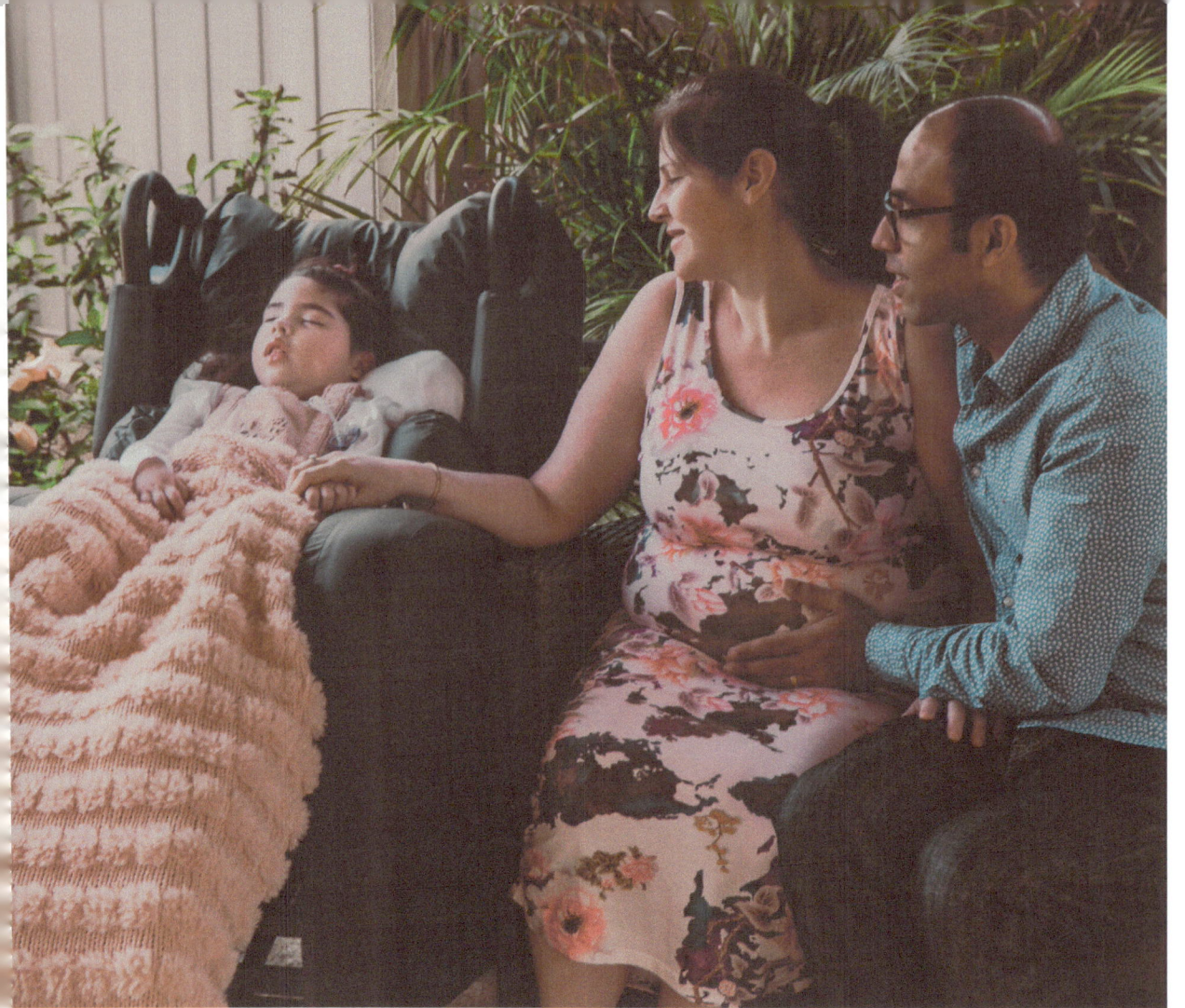

Amiya's mum, Kristy

'You always want to make sure you're doing the very best for your child – and at first, tube-feeding can be extremely daunting. Everything is so new, foreign and scary. But hang in there. After a short time you'll find yourself wondering what life was like before tube-feeding. You'll feel comfort knowing your child is getting the nutrients they need.'

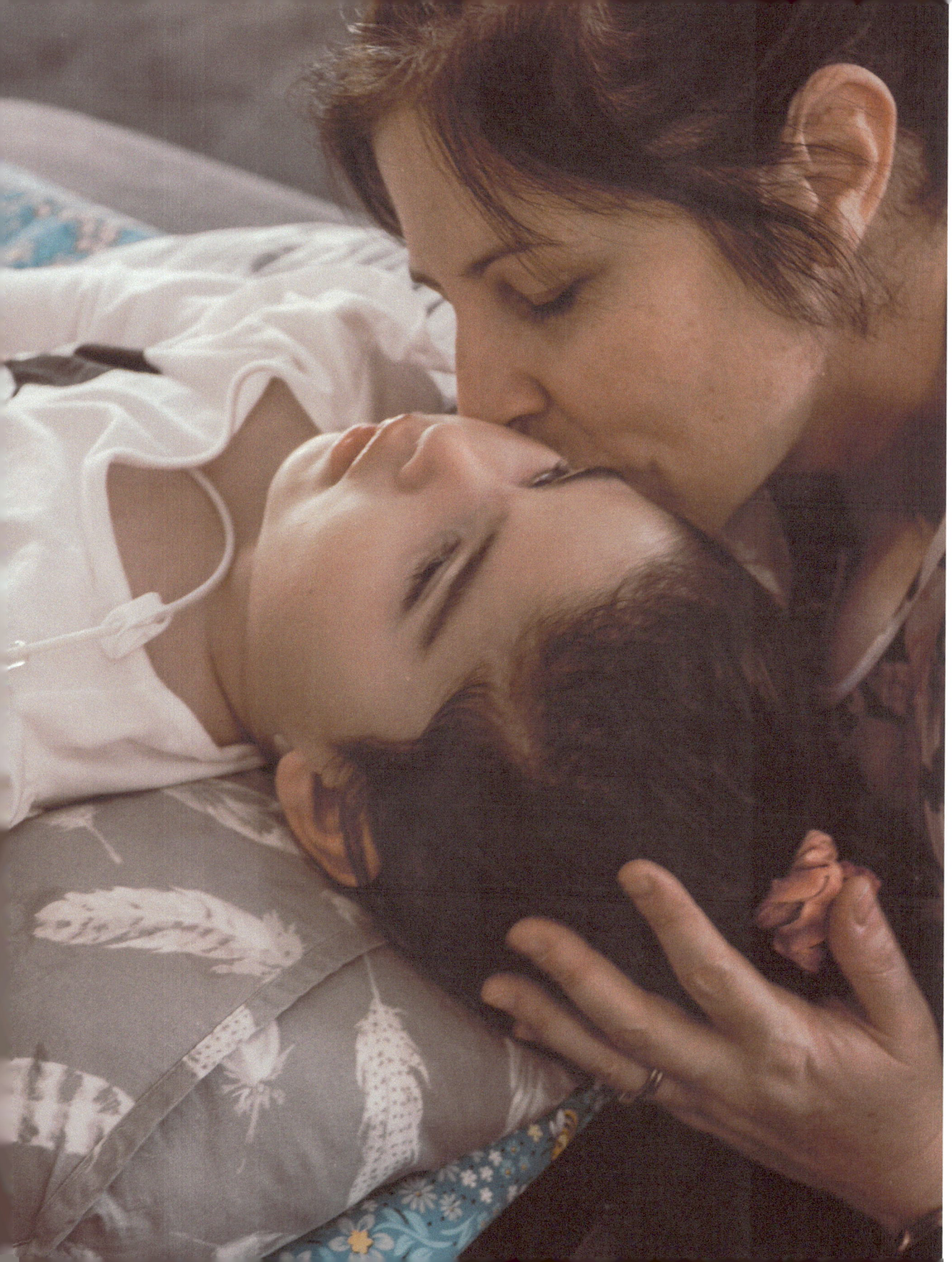

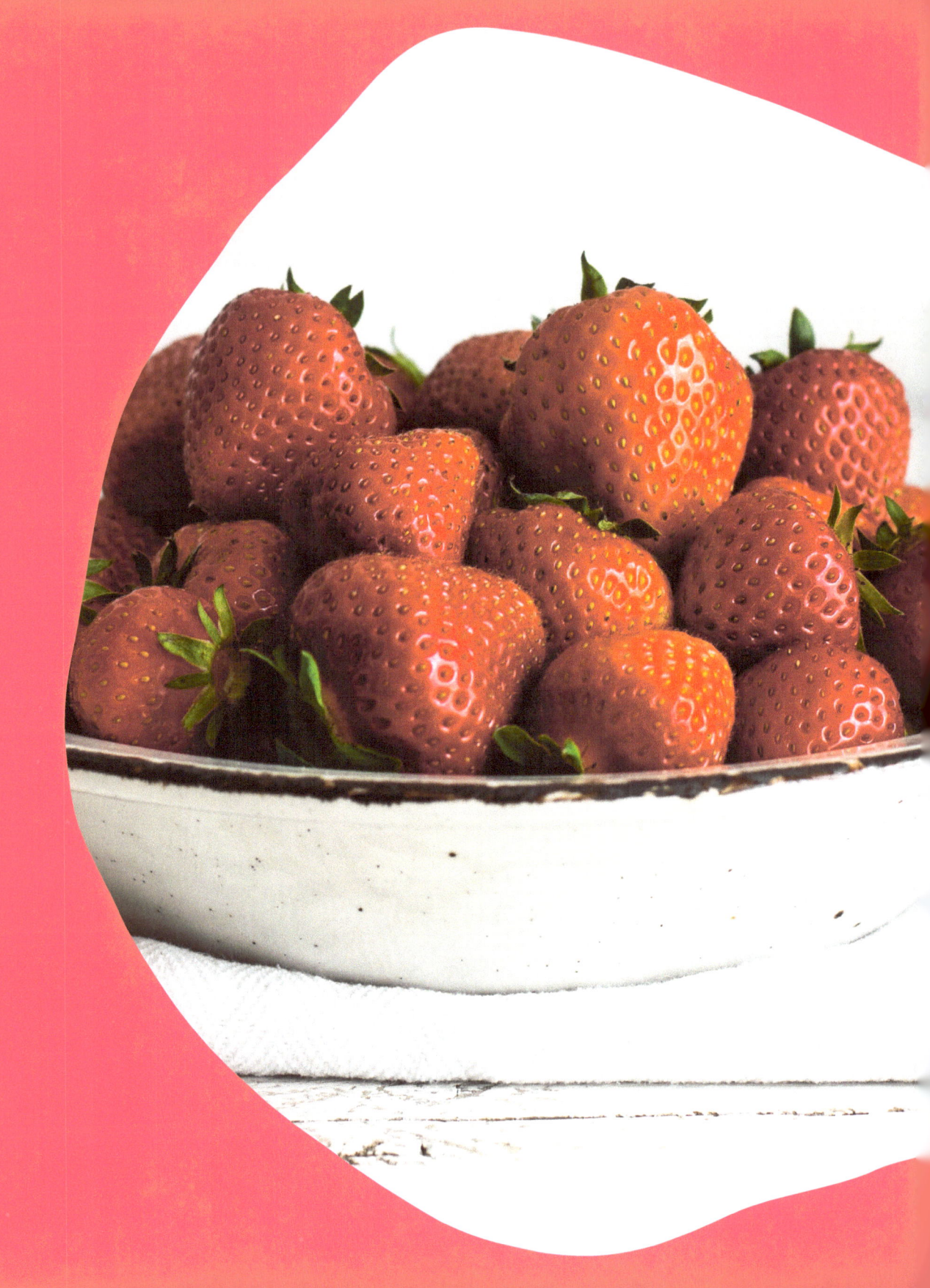

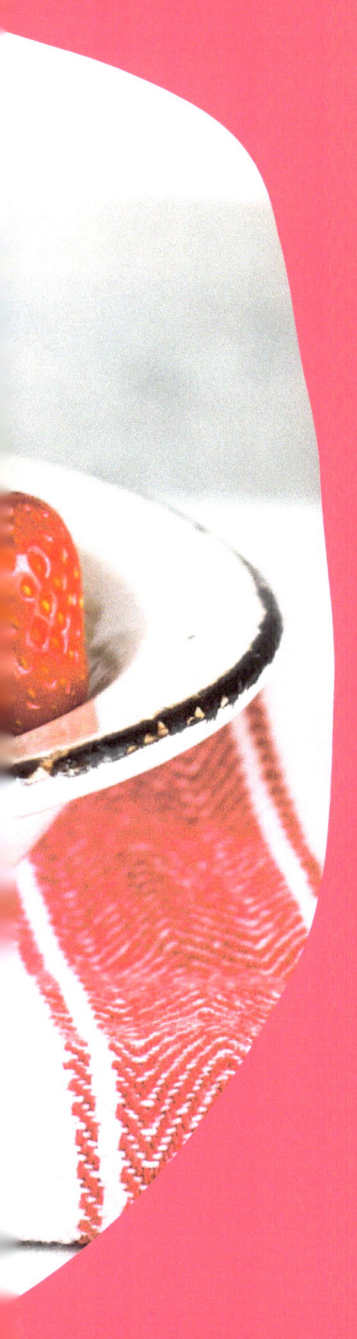

Recipes

+ **Strawberry shortcake overnight oats**

+ **Rose water milk pudding**

+ **English breakfast blend**

+ **Nachos**

+ **Peanut stew**

+ **Roasted coconutty butternut soup**

Please note: Nutritional analysis is expressed as per full batch of recipe and is a guide only.

Energy distribution (kcal/mL) is a guide only and the total volume of each batch will vary depending on the type of blender used, cooking methods and the type of ingredients used.

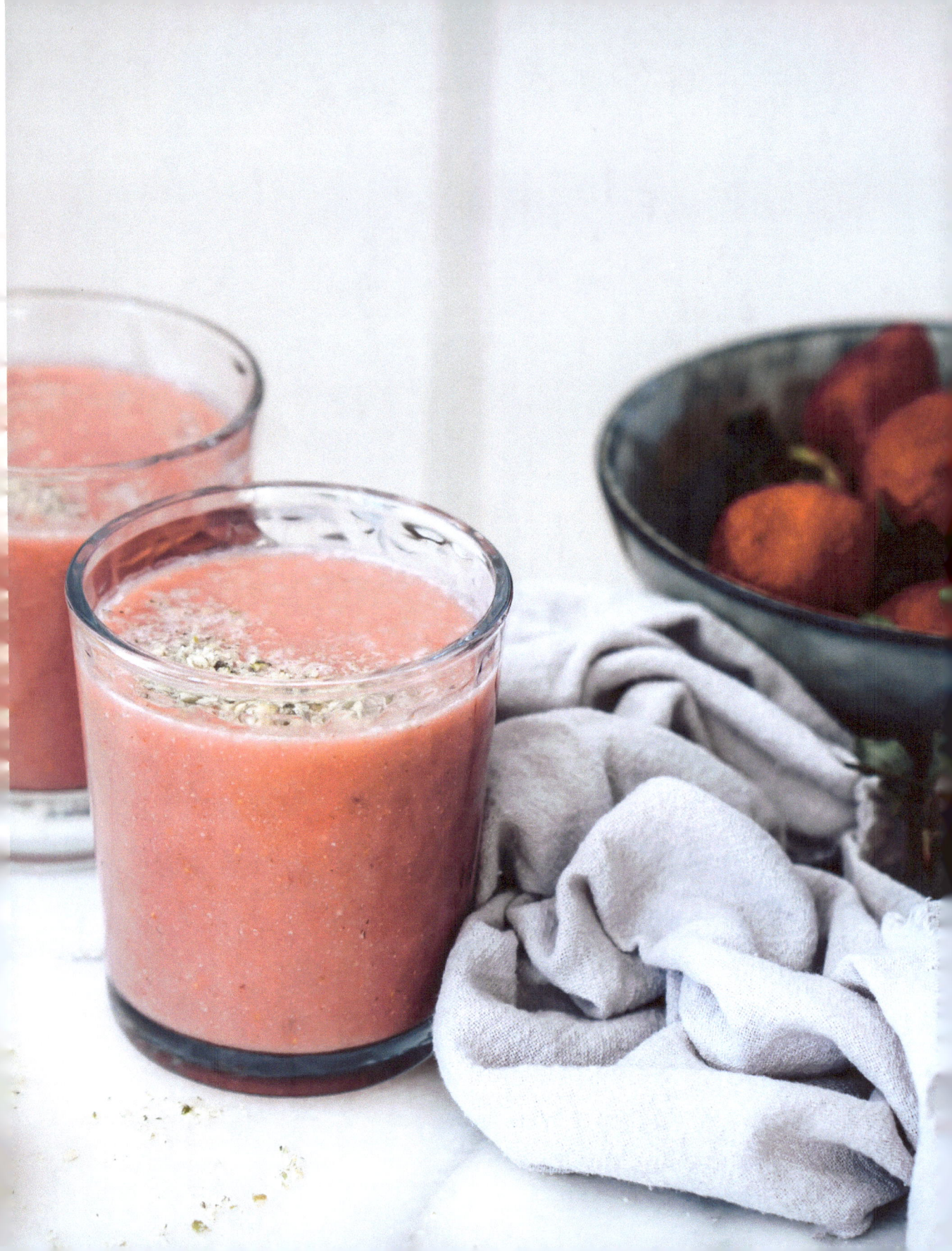

/ recipes

Hilarie Dreyer's strawberry shortcake overnight oats

Overnight oats are great for packing in nutrients and calories, and you can easily vary the ingredients. You can prep them in 10 minutes or less and in the morning will have soft food that blends easily, even if you don't have a high-tech blender.

What I love most about overnight oats for blended diets is that busy parents can also make some for themselves to eat as well. Mornings can be hectic, so having something to easily grab and blend while also being able to nourish yourself with no extra effort is a game-changer. I'm all about making the blending process as easy as possible and overnight oats are perfect for this.

Ingredients

- ⅓ **cup dry oats**
- ¾ **cup whole milk**
- ¼ **cup cottage cheese, 4% fat**
- ¼ **cup strawberries, fresh or frozen**
- **1 tablespoon hemp hearts**
- **1 ½ tablespoons honey**

Method

1. Add the dry oats, whole milk, cottage cheese, hemp hearts and honey to a jar or container with a lid, then stir together.
2. Add sliced strawberries to the top and put on the lid. Place in the fridge overnight (or for at least 4-6 hours).
3. Next morning, spoon out the overnight oats into a blender and blend until the mixture is smooth and without any lumps. This should take about 60 seconds, but it may be longer depending on your blender. Aim for a thin pancake batter consistency. Strain through a sieve if required to remove lumps. It should make up to a volume of around 420ml.

Nutrition

- **490kcal, 22g protein, 7g fibre, 2mg iron, 1.3kcal/ml**

Read Hilarie's story on page 50

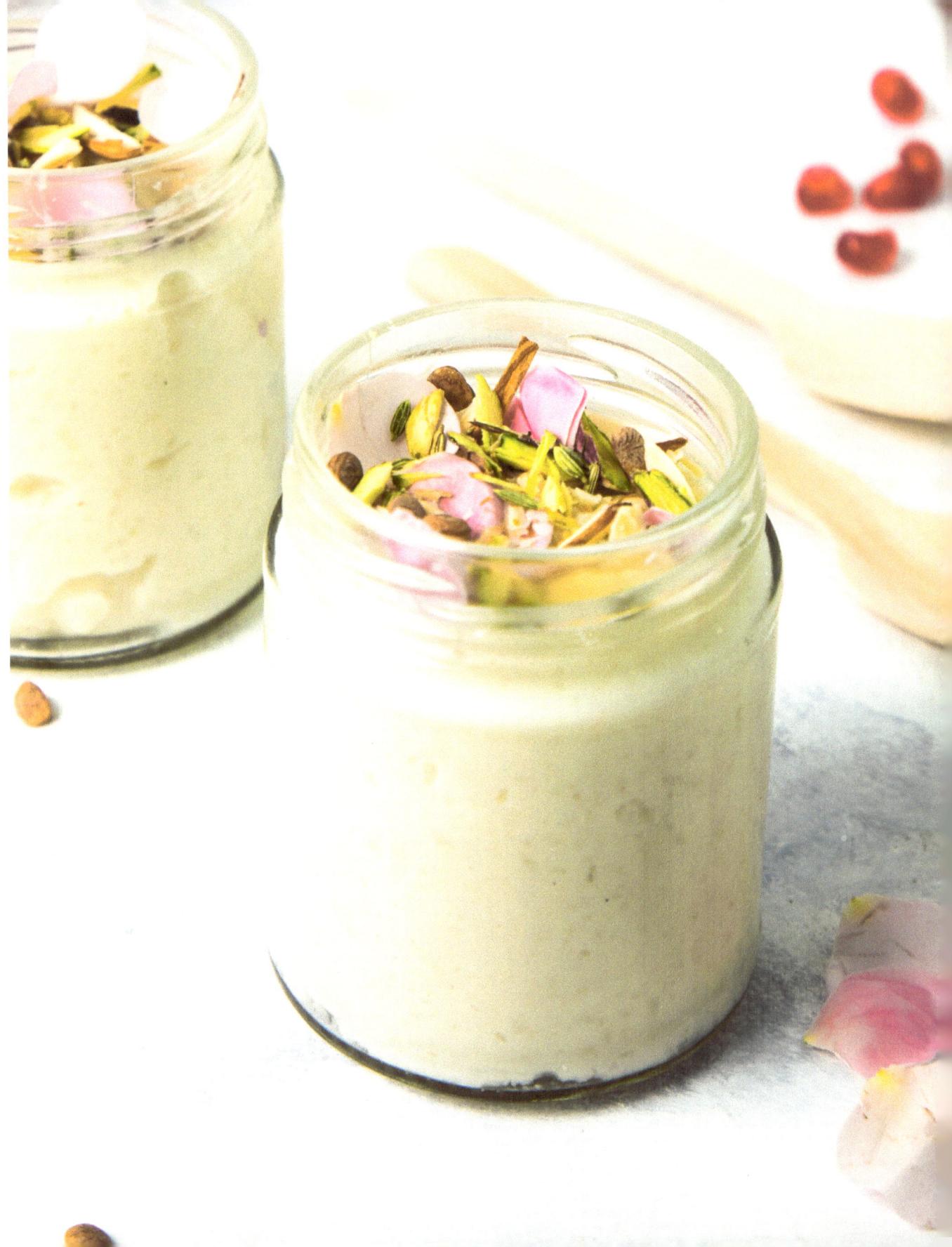

/ recipes

Lina Breik's rose water milk pudding (mahalabiya)

Ingredients

Rose water rice pudding

- 3 ¼ cups whole milk
- ¾ cup heavy whipping cream
- ½ cup granulated sugar
- ½ cup corn starch/flour
- 2 teaspoons orange blossom water
- 1 teaspoon rose water

Rose syrup topping

- 2 tablespoons rose syrup concentrate (sharbat ward)
- ¼ cup plus 2 tablespoons water
- 2 teaspoons (5g) corn starch/flour

Method

Rose water rice pudding

1. In a medium saucepan, off the heat, whisk together the milk, cream, sugar and corn starch until well combined and the corn starch has dissolved completely without any visible lumps.
2. Set the saucepan over medium-high heat and bring to a boil, whisking constantly. Continue to boil for a few more seconds until the mixture thickens and large bubbles form around the surface.
3. Remove from the heat and whisk in the orange blossom and rose waters.
4. To have through the feeding tube, pour into cups and leave to cool at room temperature (roughly 20 minutes) then syringe into your feeding tube*.
5. To eat through the mouth, pour into cups and refrigerate uncovered until the surface has begun to set (about 20 minutes). Meanwhile, prepare the rose syrup topping.

Ideal consistency for pumps/gravity feeding is smoothie. Ideal consistency for syringe feeding is ketchup. Avoid thinning the dessert with water. Add more milk to thin.

Rose syrup topping

1. In a very small saucepan, off the heat, whisk together the rose syrup concentrate, water and corn starch until well combined.
2. Set the saucepan over medium-high heat and bring to a boil, whisking constantly, until the mixture thickens and large bubbles form around the surface.
3. Remove from the heat and spoon a thin layer of the rose topping over the surface of each pudding cup, tilting the cup to cover evenly.
4. Refrigerate until set and cold – about 2 hours or up to overnight.

Nutrition

- 1950kcal, 32g protein, 1g fibre, 1mg iron, 1.5kcal/ml

Read Lina's story in Issue One of The Blend and catch her in this issue on page 12

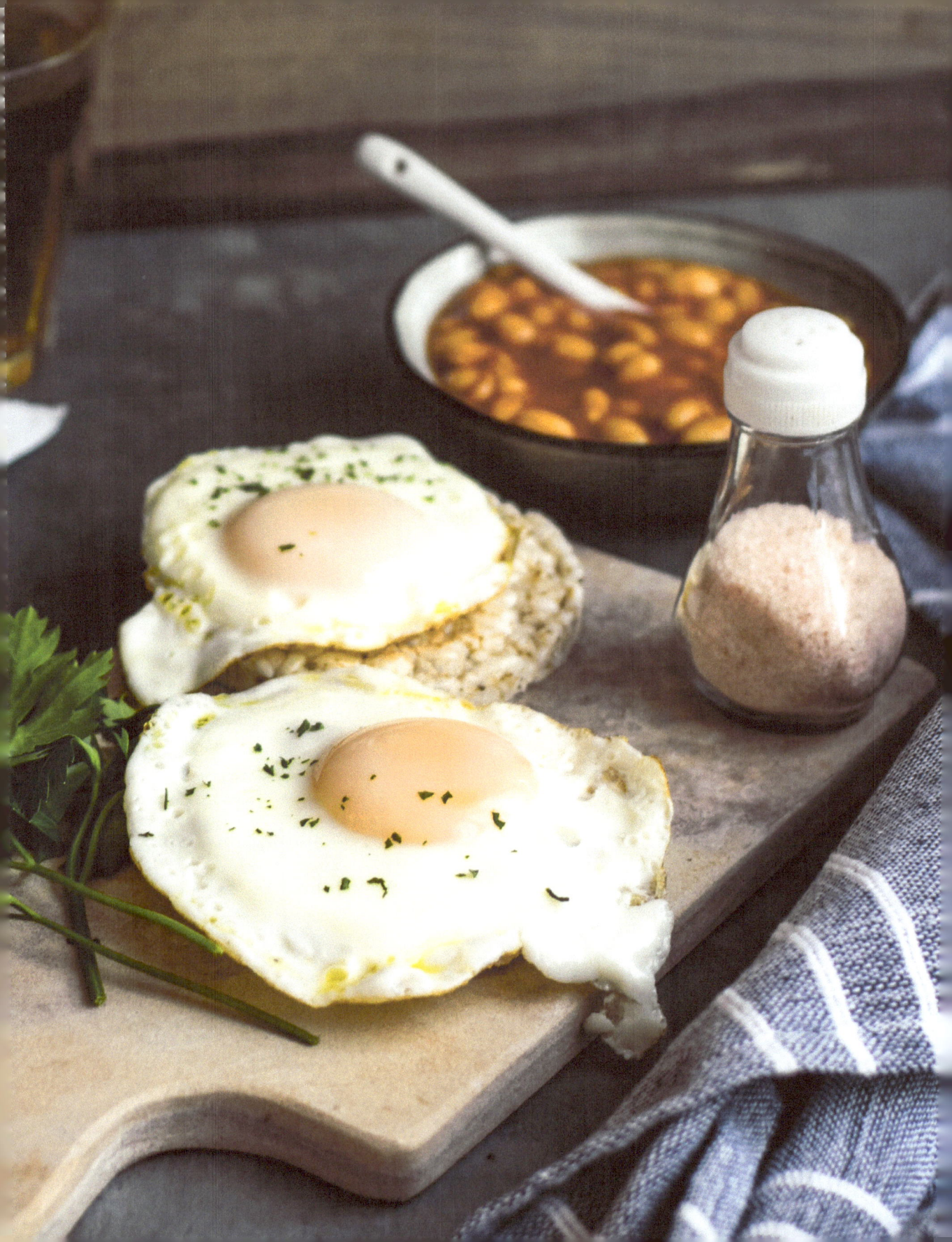

/ recipes

Kate Dehlsen's English breakfast blend

Ingredients

- 3 tablespoons baked beans
- 70g vegetable puree
- ¼ avocado
- 1 egg, scrambled well in 1 teaspoon of butter
- 150ml dairy, almond or soy milk
- 1 teaspoon coconut oil

Method

1. Combine all ingredients in a blender and blitz thoroughly until smooth.
2. Add more milk if needed. It should make up to a volume of around 350ml.
3. Strain out any lumps with a sieve.

Nutrition

- 360kcal, 15.5g protein, 6g fibre, 1.7mg iron, 1kcal/ml

Catch-up with dietitian Kate Dehlsen

'I'm excited to be involved in *The Blend* magazine Issue Two, especially seeing how popular and valuable the first edition was. I continue to be busy with providing support to children and their families with tube-feeding, via formula and blenderised diets (or both).

'Associate Professor Usha Krishnan (meet Usha on page 54) Dr Steven Leach, Neha Chandrasekar and I have recently published a study exploring clinical and nutritional outcomes between children on blended tube-feed diets and formula tube-feeds. I'm getting ready for Easter and coming up with some new blends featuring seafood, hot cross buns and Easter eggs. Wish me luck!'

Read Kate's story in The Blend Issue One

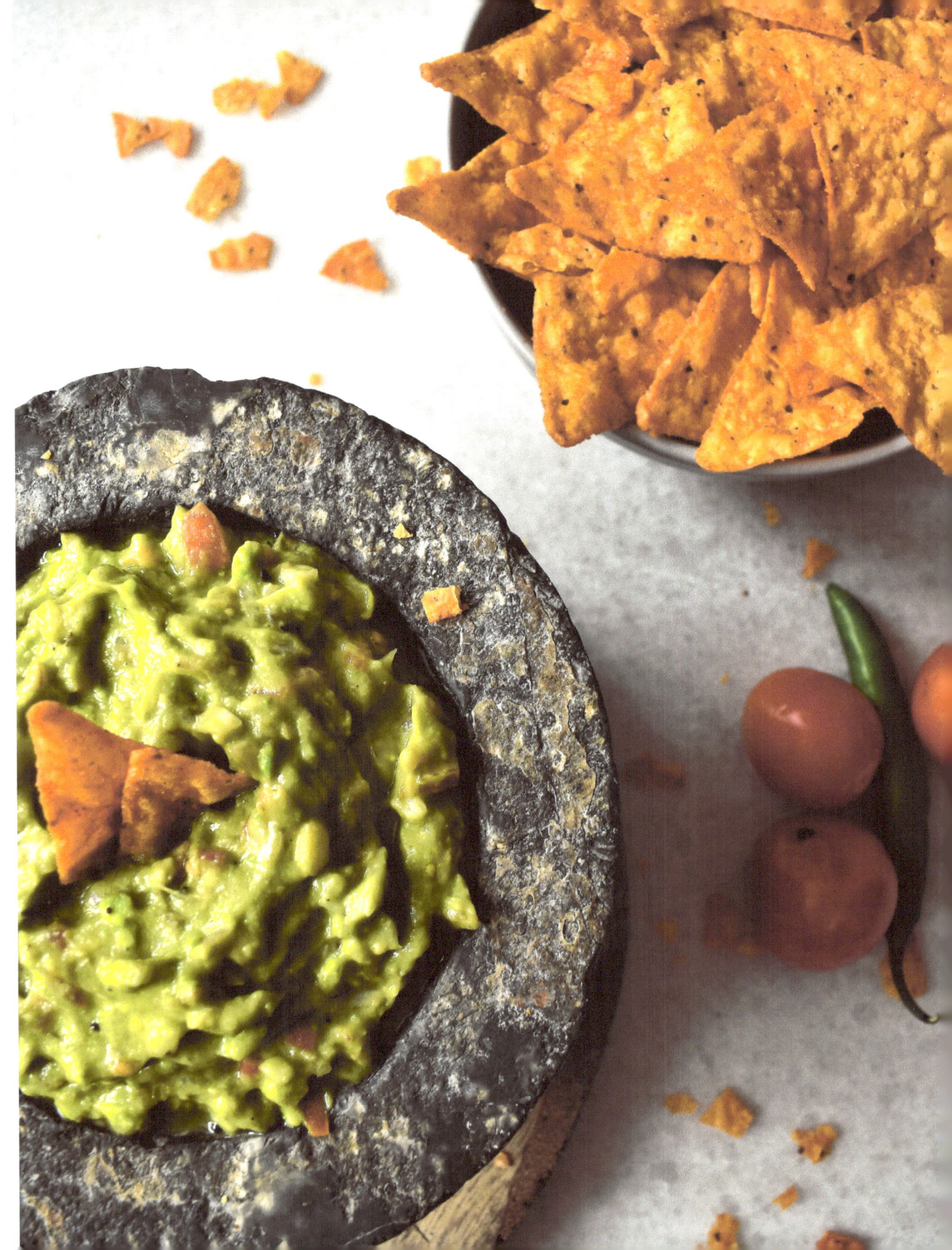

/ recipes

Sarah Thomas's nachos blend

Ingredients

- **500g corn chips**
- **1 cup grated cheese**
- **500ml chicken stock**
- **Sour cream (optional)**

Mince mix

- **1 medium-sized onion, diced**
- **500g beef mince**
- **300g jar of mild salsa**
- **1 teaspoon smoked paprika**
- **Chilli, finely chopped (optional)**

Fresh salsa

- **1 small red onion, finely chopped**
- **Small bunch of coriander, leaves and stems, chopped**
- **4 medium-sized ripe tomatoes or 8 cherry tomatoes, chopped**
- **20ml red wine vinegar**

Guacamole

- **2 tablespoons of fresh salsa mix**
- **1 large avocado**
- **Salt and pepper**
- **Lime juice (optional)**

Method

1. Preheat the oven to 220C, fan 200C, gas 7.
2. Dice onion. Add 15ml of olive oil to the pan and sauté the onion until translucent.
3. Add the mince and fry until browned.
4. Add mild salsa.
5. Add paprika and chilli (if you want it spicy).
6. Stir for 5 mins. Remove from the heat.
7. To make the fresh salsa, mix tomatoes, red onion, coriander and red wine vinegar together in a separate bowl. Set aside in the fridge until needed.
8. Spoon out 2-3 tablespoons of the fresh salsa into another bowl. Mash in the avocados to make guacamole. Season with salt and pepper. Add lime juice, if you like.
9. Pile and layer up the chips, mince and cheese on a large baking tray, scatter over remaining cheese and bake for 10-12 minutes until toasted and the cheese is bubbling.
10. Spoon over dollops of the guacamole, salsa and extra coriander.
11. Spoon sour cream over the top.
12. Blend with 500ml of chicken stock per portion (this makes 6 portions). Add more stock if needed for desired texture.

Nutrition

- **900kcal, 14.4g protein, 5g fibre, 25mg iron, 1.4kcal/ml**

Read Sarah's story in Issue One of The Blend and catch up with her in this issue on page 24

the blend.

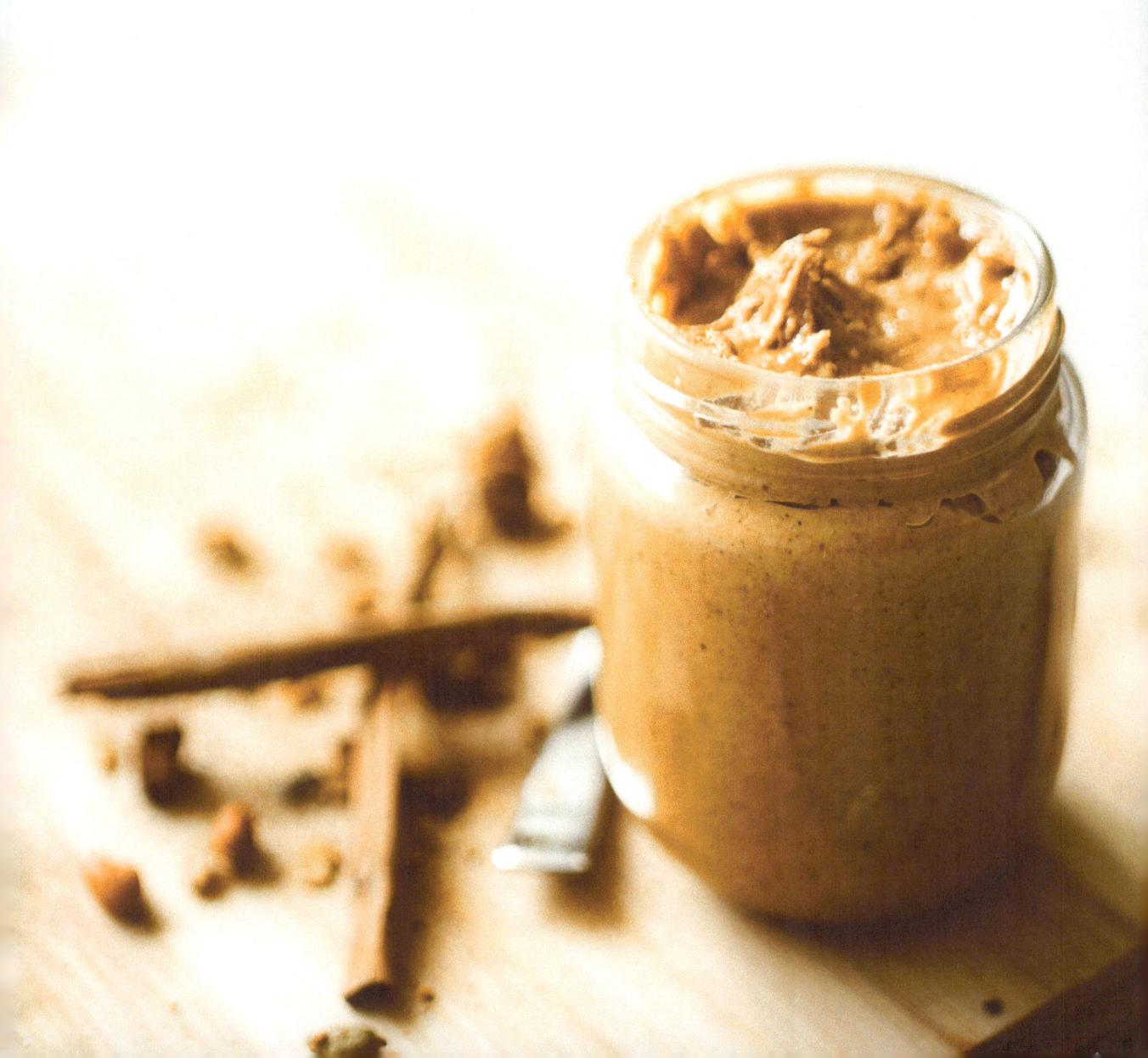

/ recipes

Claire Kariya's African peanut stew

Ingredients

- 1 cup sweet potatoes, peeled, chopped and steamed
- ½ cup boiled red lentils (cook from dry or use canned)
- ½ cup vegetable broth
- ½ cup water
- 2 tablespoons smooth peanut butter (or any nut or seed butter)
- 1 tablespoon raw white onion, chopped (optional)
- Pinch of ground cinnamon (optional)

Method

1. Blend all ingredients together. Add more broth or milk if a thinner consistency is desired. Garnish with a sprinkle of cinnamon. Makes about 475ml.
2. To enjoy by mouth, heat in a saucepan, season with salt and pepper.

Nutrition

- 505kcal, 2.1g protein, 15g fibre, 4.5mg iron, 1.1kcal/ml

Catch-up with dietitian and tube-feeding expert Claire Kariya

'I'm excited to see that blended diets continue to grow in popularity and this tube-feeding option seems to be more accepted by healthcare practitioners. There have been new published guidelines for dietitians and eight new research publications just in the past year. We're definitely finally at a place where no one can say "there isn't enough research on blenderised tube-feeding to know that it's safe". We have plenty of research showing that blending is a safe and effective tube-feeding option.

'I continue to be busy with my Natural Tube Feeding work. Last year I launched my online course for tube-fed people and their families to learn how to blend by watching a series of videos. Now I'm working on an informative webinar for dietitians who are interested in including blending in their practice.'

Read Claire's story in The Blend Issue One

- naturaltubefeeding.com
- @naturaltubefeeding
- Natural Tube Feeding

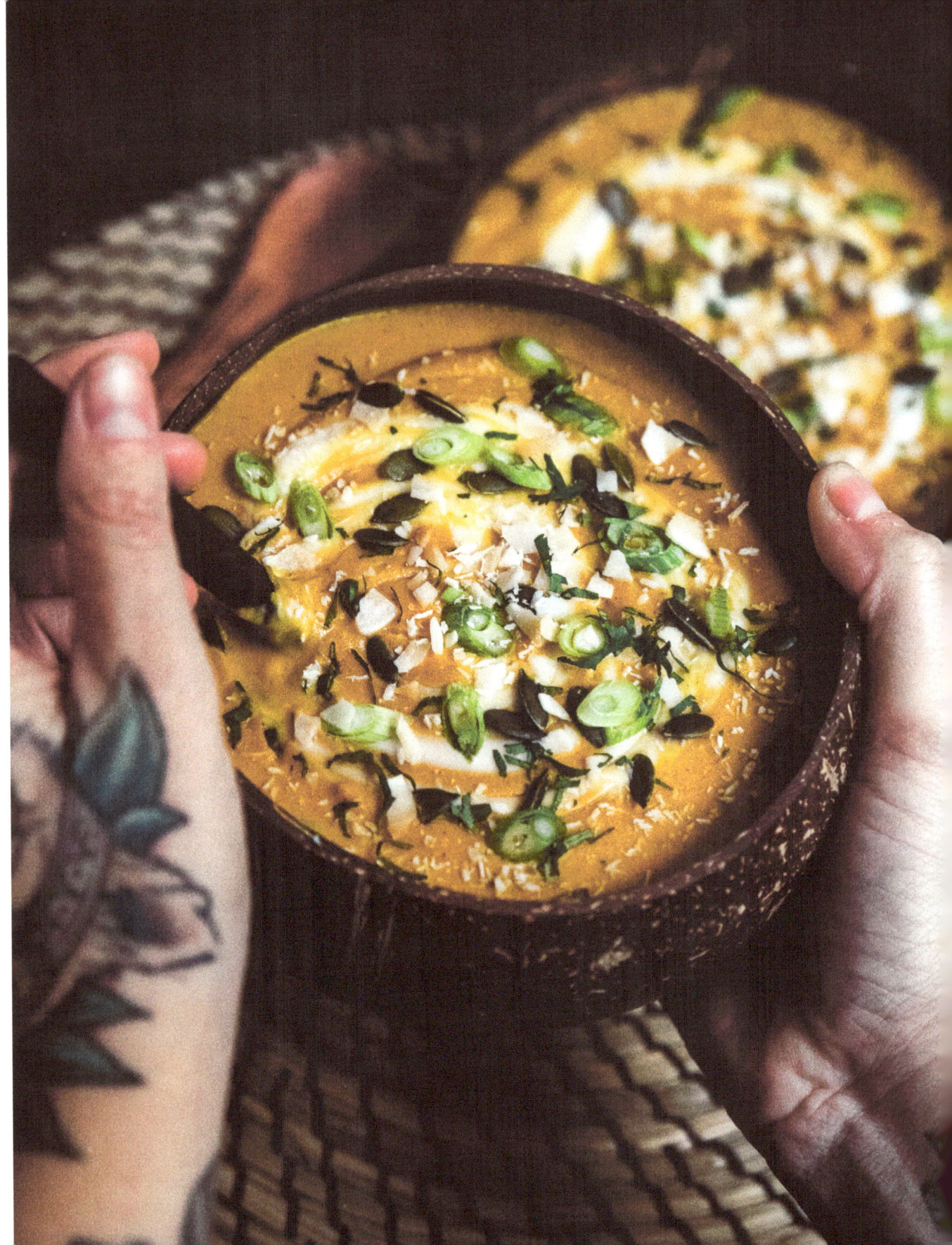

/ recipes

Loretta Harmes' roasted coconutty butternut squash soup

This soup is so velvety smooth, slightly spiced with cumin, coriander and ginger along with lime, tamari, coconut milk and almond butter for a Thai hint.

Perfect as a batch cook-and-freeze recipe which can also double up as a sauce for a quick and filling main meal. Add some of the soup to cooked onions, peppers, broccoli, spinach, chickpeas or chicken (or whatever you have lurking in the fridge) and serve it with some quinoa or rice and you've got yourself a banger!

Ingredients

- **1 large butternut squash (600g cooked flesh)**
- **1 onion, diced**
- **2 large garlic cloves, minced**
- **½ tablespoon ginger, minced**
- **400ml tin full-fat coconut milk**
- **1½ tablespoons almond butter or peanut butter**
- **¾ teaspoon cumin**
- **¾ teaspoon ground coriander**
- **½ tablespoon maple syrup**
- **1 tablespoon soy sauce**
- **1 tablespoon lime juice**
- **2 teaspoons coconut oil**
- **½ teaspoon Himalayan salt**

Optional toppings
(wouldn't recommend blending these)

- **Toasted pumpkin seeds**
- **Coconut yoghurt**
- **Coconut chips**
- **Desiccated coconut**
- **Spring onions**
- **Fresh coriander**

Method

1. Preheat the oven to 180C. Cut the butternut pumpkin in half, scrape out the seeds. Brush with oil and bung the halves on to a baking tray. Roast for around one hour or until the pumpkin flesh is completely soft. This can be done in advance or used straight from the oven.
2. In a saucepan, fry onions in the coconut oil until soft and translucent (about 5 mins). Add in the spices, garlic and ginger, cook for 2 minutes stirring regularly.
3. Add in the remaining ingredients, bring to the boil and simmer for a couple of minutes.
4. Pour into a blender and blitz until smooth. You may have to do this in batches to achieve a velvet-smooth texture.
5. If eating straight away, add back into the pan and heat until warm.

Nutrition

- **1295kcal, 31g protein, 20g fibre, 8.7mg iron, 1kcal/ml**

Read Loretta's story on page 66

Directory

A collection of products and online communities for tube-feeding.

Accessories

Tubie Fun

Celebrating feeding in a different way, Tubie Fun provides a variety of products that assist with the ease and comfort of anyone who is tube-fed. Find an interview with founder Stacey Phillips in Issue One of The Blend and a catch-up with her on page 20.

- tubiefun.com.au
- @tubiefunau
- @tubiefun

Tubie Love

After seeing how much her own son, Aidan, benefited from her handmade G-tube button pads and belts, Tammy Smith started Tubie Love. She now makes a range of accessories, straight from her kitchen table and stocks adhesive tapes from A Simple Patch.

- tubielove.com
- @tubielove
- Tubie Love

Tremendous Tubies

Jessica Hall started making tubie pouches for her son so he could get around without his NG tube dragging and getting snagged. So came Tremendous Tubies, Jessica's Etsy store where you can find a collection of adorable pouches and tubie clips for kids and adults.

- etsy.com/au/shop/tremendoustubies
- @tremendoustubies
- @Tremendous Tubies

The Travelling Tubie Project

The Travelling Tubie Project is the business of tubie mama, Chloe Turner. It offers nasogastric and oxygen tube adhesive tapes that are strong, long-lasting and suitable for all types of faces and tubes. Recently, they've added pump hangers, stickers and tubie milestone cards to the mix. Flick over to page 98 to read Chloe's story.

- tubieproject.com
- @the.travelling.tubie.project
- The Travelling Tubie Project

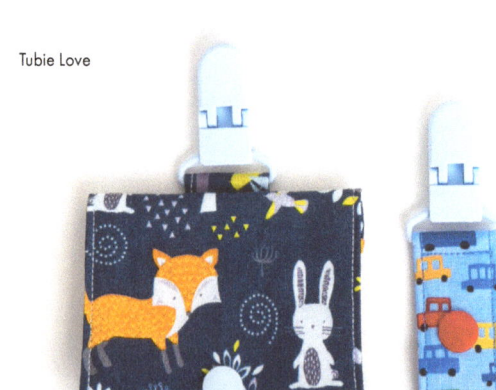

Tubie Love

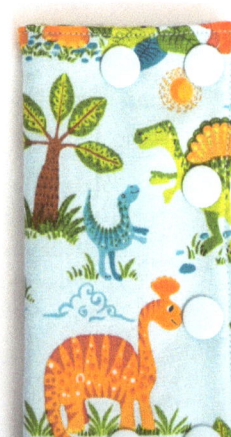

/ directory

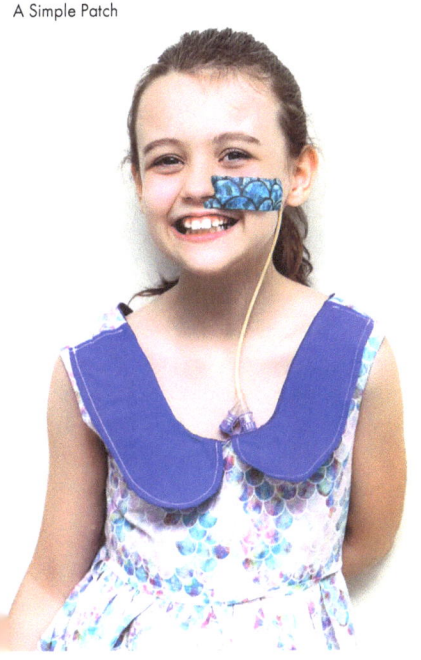

A Simple Patch

Megan Wassink's daughter uses medical devices and tubes and Megan wanted to make them look less medical. Enter A Simple Patch, an online store selling fun and firmly-sticking medical tape in a range of prints or, if you like, a custom design of your own choosing.

 asimplepatch.com
 @asimplepatch
 @asimplepatch

RockTape Rx

Kinesiology tape maker, RockTape, has a range specially designed to be gentler on skin called RockTape Rx. It's hypo-allergenic, contains no zinc oxide or latex and is water-resistant, with a wear-time of up to five days. It also comes in four kiddo and adult-friendly designs.

 rocktape.com.au
 @rocktapeaustralia
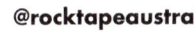 @rocktapeaustralia

The Priceless Feeding Tube Accessories

Ever found your child swimming in a lake of formula? Joshua Fast has, so he got himself a 3D-printer and crafted some solutions. Joshua's biz, The Priceless, designs and manufactures tube and button locks to prevent accidental dislocation (and to 'avoid hangry tube-feeders', as Joshua says).

 thepriceless.ca

Spewy

They're designed for kids who occasionally spew or wet their bed (so, all kids). But boy are these beauties useful for any kind of leak in the night. With its microfibre and terry towelling blend of layers and waterproof backing, a Spewy mat can absorb and contain up to two litres of liquid. Plus, they come in a range of sweet prints.

 spewy.com.au
@spewyau
 Spewy

GranuLotion

This stuff is what it says on the label – a lotion to treat granulation tissue. One that's getting two very enthusiastic thumbs-up from tube-feeders the world over. Slather it on at home and skip the silver nitrate treatments and harsh topical steroids. And if you're aiming for precision, you'll be glad to know GranuLotion now comes in a needle-tip tube.

 granulotion.com
@GranuLotion

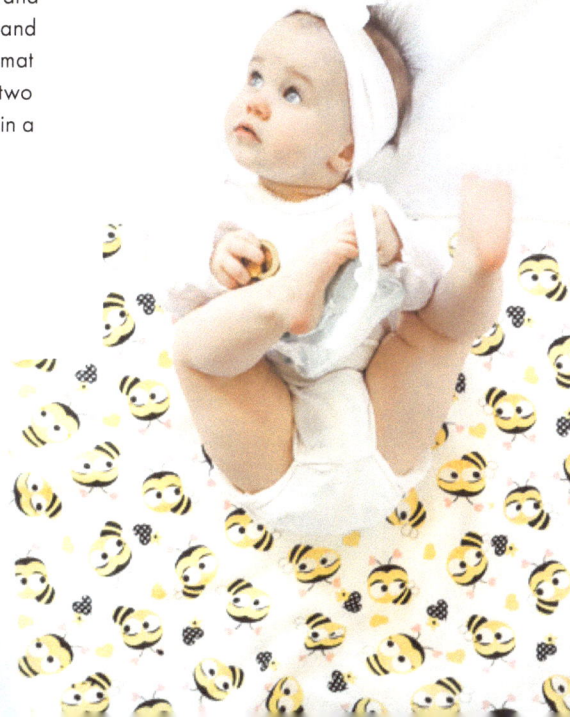

Spewy

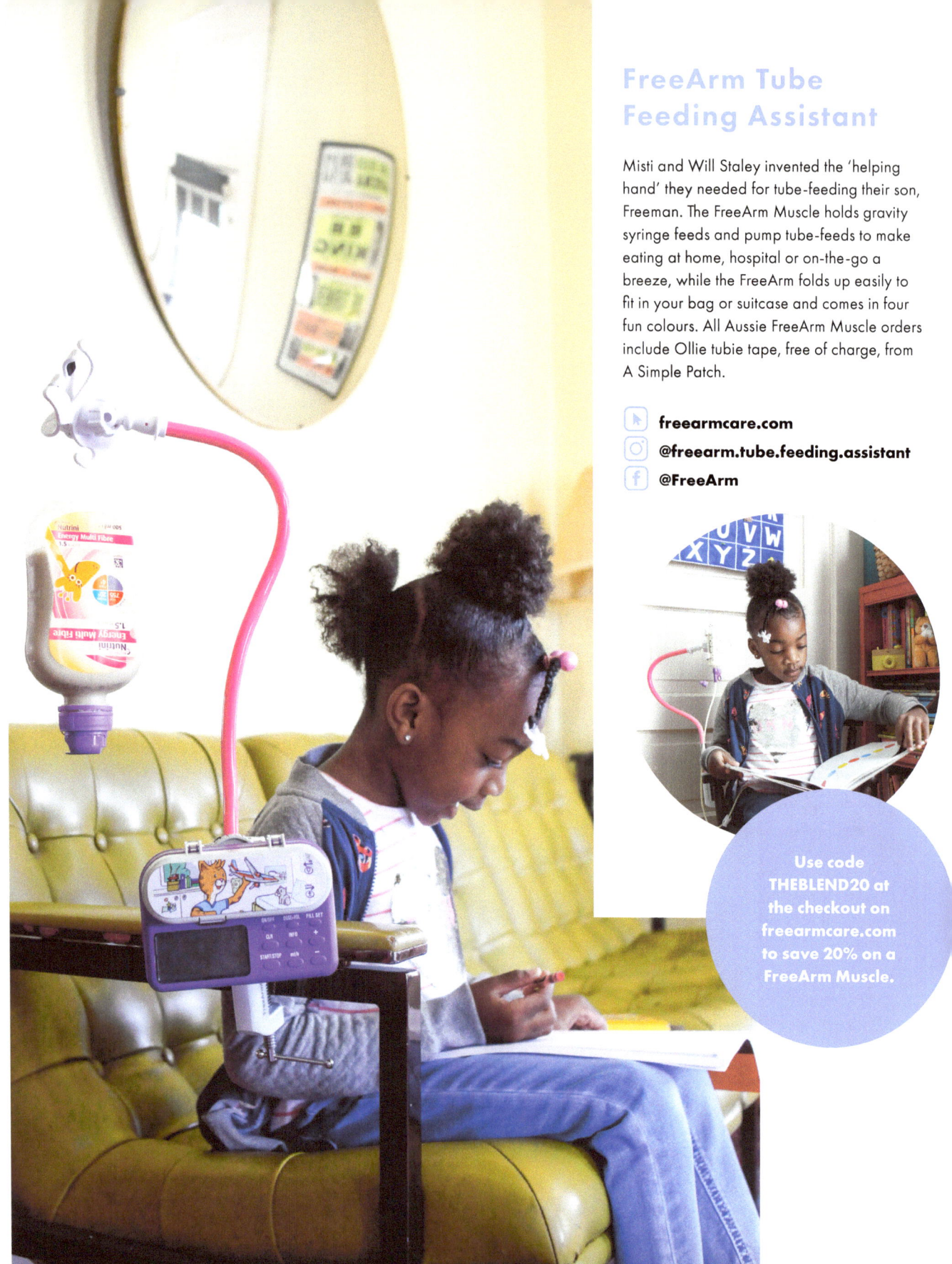

FreeArm Tube Feeding Assistant

Misti and Will Staley invented the 'helping hand' they needed for tube-feeding their son, Freeman. The FreeArm Muscle holds gravity syringe feeds and pump tube-feeds to make eating at home, hospital or on-the-go a breeze, while the FreeArm folds up easily to fit in your bag or suitcase and comes in four fun colours. All Aussie FreeArm Muscle orders include Ollie tubie tape, free of charge, from A Simple Patch.

freearmcare.com
@freearm.tube.feeding.assistant
@FreeArm

Use code **THEBLEND20** at the checkout on freearmcare.com to save 20% on a FreeArm Muscle.

Storage + Organisation

Subo – The Food Bottle

Here we have a non-squeezable, mess-free bottle made for blended feeds. This product is perfect for storing meals and, should they fancy it, a bit of self-feeding for your kid. As team Subo says, bottoms up!

- suboproducts.com.au
- @suboproducts
- @SuboProducts

Sinchies

Sinchies reusable food pouches connect directly to G-tubes for gravity feeding and can also be used with Infinity feeding pumps. They're super-lightweight – perfect for popping in a small backpack, allowing greater mobility – and are available in cute designs for the kiddos.

- sinchies.com.au
- @sinchies
- @Sinchies

Boon Grass Drying Rack

This widely used and loved bottle drying rack just happens to work a treat for syringes and other bits of tube-feeding kit. You can buy the Boon Grass Drying Rack from several Aussie/NZ retailers. Helpful hack: Dry your syringes tip-down on this one.

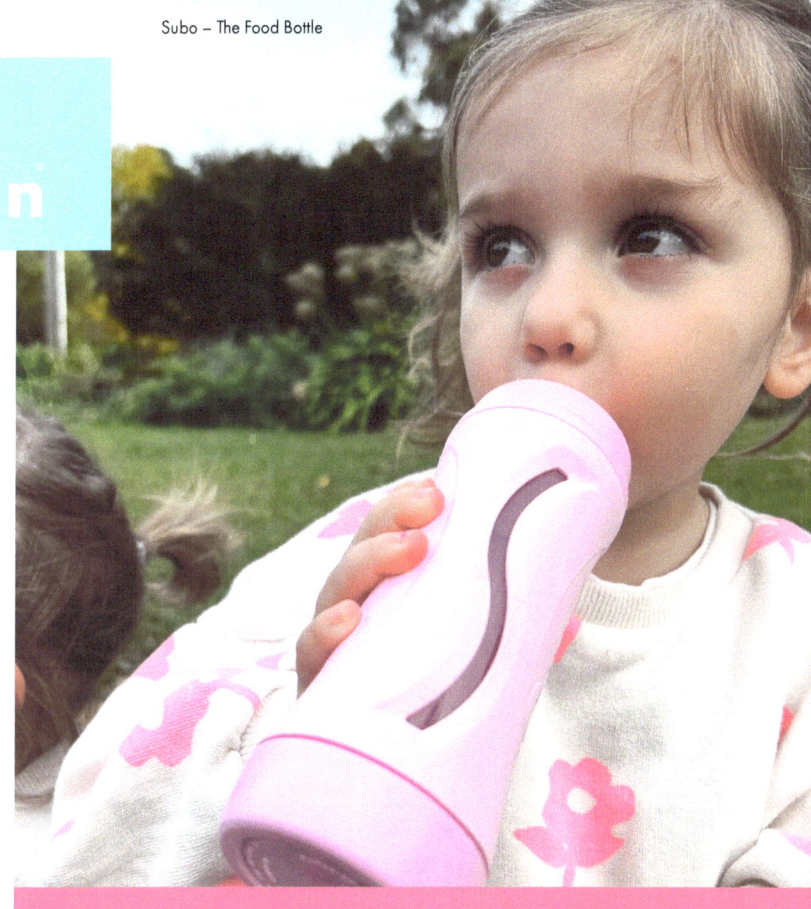

Blend feeding

Wholesome Blends

Founded by Sarah Thomas (who you can catch up with on page 24), Wholesome Blends is a maker of healthy, high-calorie meals that are a godsend for tubie families on the go. Pantry-stable and stored in a pouch, their pork, chicken and vegetarian blends have a whopping, year-long shelf-life – and Sarah's got a range of new recipes in development.

- wholesomeblends.com.au
- @wholesomeblendsau
- @wholesomeblend

ChooMee Softsip Food Pouch Tops

ChooMee's pouch top is a reusable mouthpiece with a cap that attaches to all standard food pouch brands. It's designed to protect little mouths, but the blended-feeding community has found that you can use it to draw blended food straight out of a pouch with a syringe, mess-free.

- choomee.com
- @choomee
- @ChoomeeInc

Fashion

Whole Enteral

A nutritionally formulated meal replacement called Enrich is the debut product of Whole Enteral, the business baby of Ali Howell and speech pathologist Emily Lively (flip to page 23 to catch up with these co-founders). Nut, dairy, gluten, soy and GMO-free, Enrich is made from plant-based wholefoods and meets the Australian Food Standard for Formulated Meal Replacement.

 whole.net.au
 @whole_en
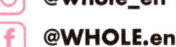 @WHOLE.en

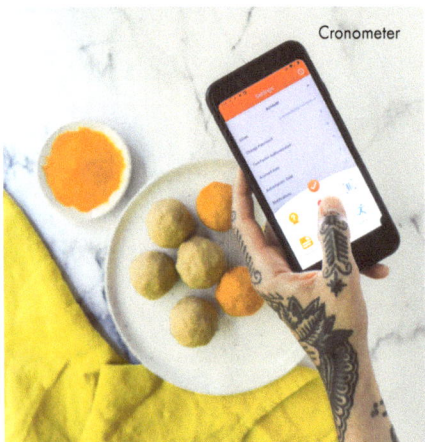
Cronometer

Cronometer

This pocket-friendly tool claims to be 'the most accurate, comprehensive nutrition tracking app on Earth'. Which could come in very handy if you're trying to keep those calories up. Tell Cronometer your blended feed ingredients and it'll let you know the exact nutritional value going in.

 cronometer.com
 @cronometer_official
 @cronometer

Ready Set Romper

These Canadian, premium bamboo fabric rompers (read: jumpsuits) have no snap fasteners, buttons or zippers, making them a go-to for medical and tubie families across the globe. Better still, every romper sold gives back to a mother in Uganda through the Tekera Resource Centre.

 readysetromper.com
 @readysetromper
 @readysetromper

StomaStoma

Darlene and Nick Abrams are the wife-and-husband duo behind the StomaStoma clothing brand and community, which started as a family effort to support their son, Owen, who has a tracheostomy and G-tube. Now with a range of cool, stoma-positive tees and onesies, Darlene and Nick say: 'Art on shirts isn't going to change the world, but we believe it can be one part of taking this overwhelming and scary situation and making it a little bit better.'

 stomastoma.com
 @hi_stomastoma
 @histomastoma

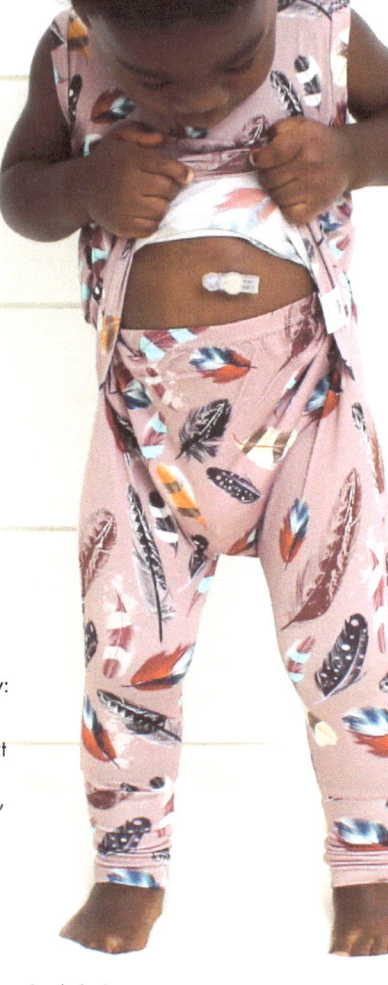
Ready Set Romper

Online Communities

- childfeeding.org
- ausee.org
- feedingtubeawareness.org
- tubefed.com.au
- BlenderizedRN Facebook group
- Feeding Tube Australia Facebook group

/ directory

Littlest Warrior

The label that trademarked 'advocate like a mother' has something to empower pretty much every family in the medical space – including some very cute Tubie Warrior onesies. Want something in a larger size? Fear not. Littlest Warrior founder Michelle Sullivan says: 'I can make them as tees, too!'

- littlestwarrior.com
- @littlest_warrior
- @littlestwarrior

Marks and Spencer Kids Easy Dressing range

Big brands are becoming more inclusive (cheers to that) and the M&S collection of adaptable apparel and accessories is, from all reports, a tube-feeding family favourite.

- marksandspencer.com/l/kids/easy-dressing

Wonsie

Wonsie was started by Sydney mum, Julie O'Donovan, when a friend of hers asked her to make a specialised bodysuit for their son who has a disability. Wonsie comes in several designs including a tummy-access range to make tube-feeding easier. These soft cotton bodysuits are available in all sizes, from toddlers all the way to large adults.

- wonsie.com.au
- @wonsie
- @wonsiekids

Books

The Abilities in Me: Tube Feeding

Written by medical mama Gemma Keir, this kids' picture book follows the story of a young girl, inspired by the UK's Chanel Murrish, who's had an NG, PEG and MIC-KEY button.

- theabilitiesinme.com
- @theabilitiesinmebookseries
- @theabilitiesinmebookseries

The Original Natural Tube Feeding Recipe eBook

Registered dietitian Claire Kariya shares 20 tried-and-tested blended meal recipes, each with their own nutritional information, in this photo-filled, downloadable ebook. Find one of her recipes on page 124.

- naturaltubefeeding.com
- @naturaltubefeeding
- @naturaltubefeeding

Easy Follow Easy Swallow: Transitioning off a PEG tube back to oral eating

This recipe book is the work of trained chef and head and neck cancer survivor Yvonne McClaren, who you can meet in Issue One of The Blend.

- yvonnemcclaren.com
- @yvonnegracemcclaren
- @nofeedingtubes

the blend.

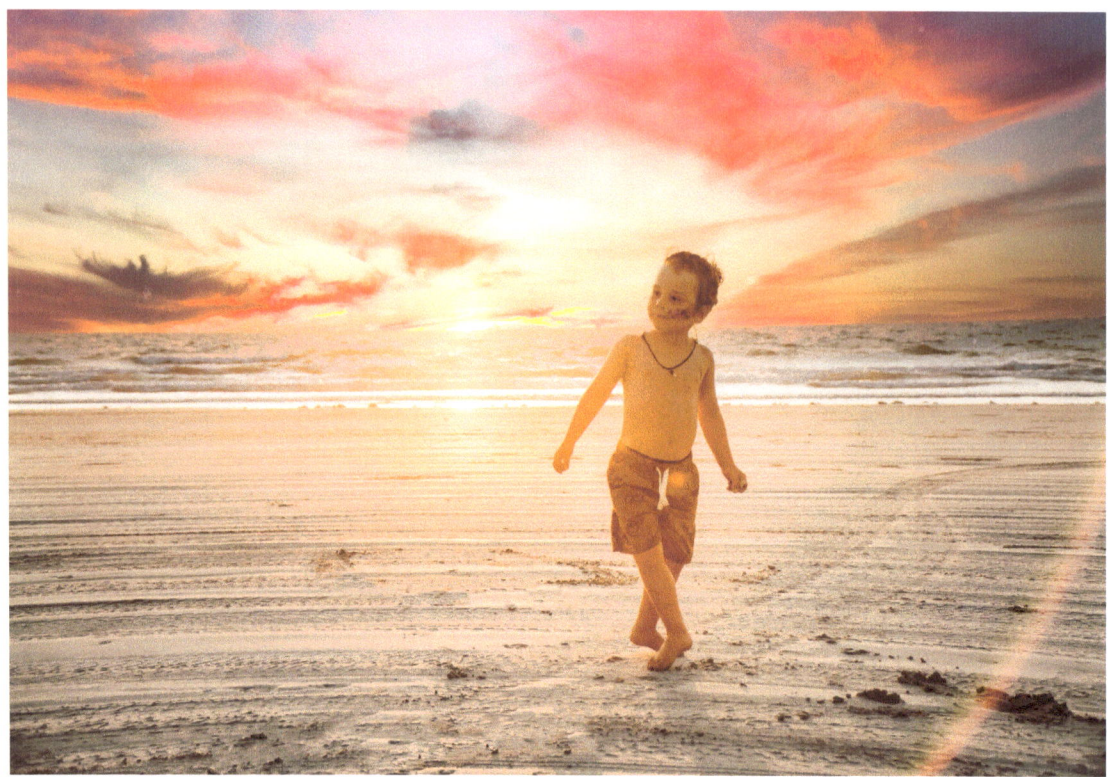

Photography: Chloe Turner / The Travelling Tubie Project

The Blend magazine is an independent publication

Founder and editor
Melanie Dimmitt
melaniedimmitt.com.au

Creative director
Edie Swan
edieswan.com

Published by
Printcraft Pty Ltd

Legal stuff
No part of this publication may be reproduced by any means without prior written permission of the editor. Views expressed within The Blend magazine are not necessarily those of the editor.

theblendmag.com

FINALLY, A WHOLE MEAL FOR YOUR TUBE

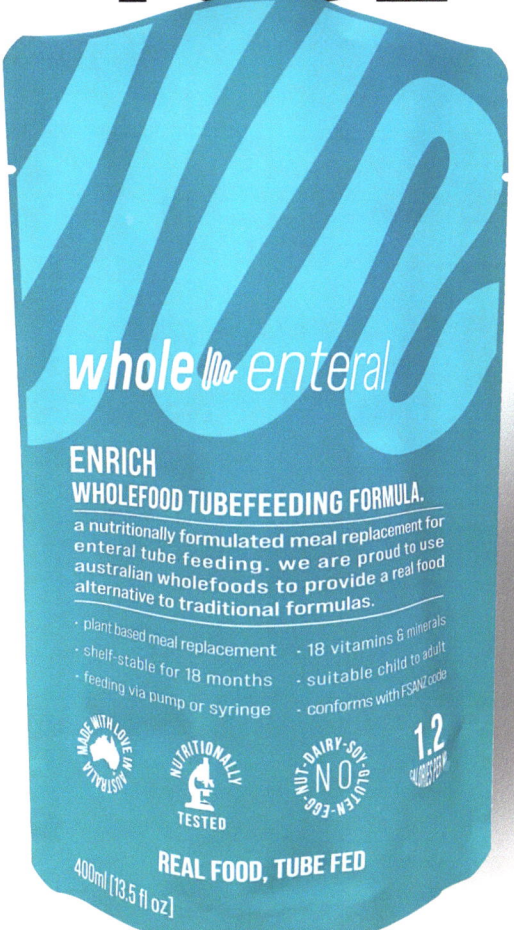

whole enteral

whole.net.au

scan to learn more

www.ingramcontent.com/pod-product-compliance
Lightning Source LLC
Chambersburg PA
CBHW050739110526
44590CB00002B/22